Pilates

Mat

Training

By Shirley Archer, J.D., M.A.

A Guide for

Fitness

Professionals

from the

American

Council

on Exercise®

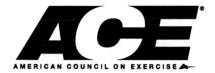

AMERICAN COUNCIL ON EXERCISE

ISBN: 1-58518-915-4
Library of Congress Control Number: 2004113367

Distributed by:
American Council on Exercise
P.O. Box 910449
San Diego, CA 92191-0449
(858) 279-8227
(858) 279-8064 (FAX)
www.ACEfitness.org

Managing Editor: Daniel J. Green
Technical Editor: Cedric X. Bryant, Ph.D.
Design & Production: Karen McGuire
Director of Publications: Christine J. Ekeroth
Assistant Editor: Jennifer Schiffer
Index: Bonny McLaughlin
Models: Shirley Archer, Monica Bowditch, &
Fran Philip
Photography: Dennis Dal Covey

Acknowledgments:
Thanks to the entire American Council on Exercise staff for their support and guidance
through the process of creating this manual.

NOTICE

The fitness industry is ever-changing. As new research and clinical experience broaden our knowledge,
changes in programming and standards are required. The authors and the publisher of this work have
checked with sources believed to be reliable in their efforts to provide information that is complete and
generally in accord with the standards accepted at the time of publication. However, in view of the
possibility of human error or changes in industry standards, neither the authors nor the publisher nor
any other party who has been involved in the preparation or publication of this work warrants that the
information contained herein is in every respect accurate or complete, and they are not responsible for
any errors or omissions or the results obtained from the use of such information. Readers are encouraged to confirm the information contained herein with other sources.

Published by:
Healthy Learning Books & Videos
P.O. Box 1828
Monterey, CA 93942
(888) 229-5745
(831) 372-6075 (Fax)
www.healthylearning.com

P05-003

Kevin A. Bowen is the co-founder and president/CEO of the Pilates Method Alliance, an international not-for-profit professional association dedicated to the teachings of Joseph H. and Clara Pilates. Bowen has been actively involved in the Pilates community for more than 10 years, is the author of *The Absolute Beginner's Guide to the Pilates Method,* and has been featured on CNN and the Discovery Channel.

Elizabeth Larkam, in her 19 years as a Pilates professional, has designed programs for fitness, dance, sports, rehabilitation, and academic settings. She is certified in Feldenkrais, Gyrokinesis, and Gyrotonic exercise and is the director of Pilates & Beyond for Western Athletic Clubs. Larkam has headed the Pilates program at the Center for Sports Medicine, Saint Francis Memorial Hospital, and taught exercise and sports science at the University of San Francisco. She created the Pilates Allegro workout series, the Pilates Mat with Roller & Ring program, Reebok Core Pilates, BOSU Pilates, and PilatesPerformance. Larkam is an American Council on Exercise spokesperson and Reebok Master Trainer.

REVIEWERS

CONTENTS

The American Council on Exercise (ACE) is pleased to introduce *Pilates Mat Training,* a guide for fitness professionals. Consumer demand for Pilates mat training continues to grow and fitness professionals are recognizing the value of incorporating Pilates mat exercise into a comprehensive training program. The intent of this book is to educate and give guidance to personal trainers that wish to train clients using Pilates mat exercises in a one-on-one setting, as well as group fitness instructors teaching Pilates mat classes or incorporating some Pilates mat exercises into other types of classes. The purpose of this manual is to provide a brief introduction and overview, a description of the principles and application of Pilates mat exercises, and an exercise sampling. Safety issues are also highlighted. However, the material presented in this book is not intended to confer competency regarding the discipline of Pilates. As with all areas of fitness, education is a continual process. ACE recognizes this is a broad subject requiring serious study and we encourage you to use the References and Suggested Reading and to obtain appropriate training to further your knowledge and skills.

INTRODUCTION

Introduction to Pilates Mat Training

CHAPTER ONE

History

Joseph Hubertus Pilates created the Pilates method of exercise at the beginning of the 20th century. Born in 1880 near Dusseldorf, Germany, Pilates suffered a sickly childhood with asthma, rickets, and rheumatic fever. To improve his health as a youth, he turned to physical training and pursued diving, skiing, gymnastics, boxing, and bodybuilding. By age 14, his physique was so well developed that he worked as a model for anatomical charts. He pursued a varied career as a boxer, fitness trainer, and circus performer, among other activities.

In 1912, Pilates moved to England, where he had many jobs including self-defense instructor to detectives at Scotland Yard. When World War I erupted, the British government labeled Pilates as an enemy alien and placed him in an internment camp. While imprisoned, he provided exercise training to other internees and worked in a hospital to help bedridden patients. He used his time to develop physical conditioning methods to rehabilitate these patients and created training equipment from hospital beds, using springs to facilitate exercise. These inventions formed the basis for the now popular reformer, which still resembles a cot, and for the trapeze table, sometimes called the "Cadillac," which looks like a table with hanging springs and bars.

In 1926, Pilates immigrated to New York and opened a training studio with his wife, Clara, whom he met on the ship as he traveled to America. The Pilates' clientele included many prominent ballet and modern dancers of the era. Today, Pilates exercises remain a staple of dance conditioning.

Pilates passed away in 1967 at the age of 87, possibly as a result of smoke inhalation suffered during a fire in the building where his studio was located. During his lifetime, Pilates was known to be very protective of his exercise method and only trained a handful of apprentices to help with instruction at his studio. Pilates did not designate any one individual to be the sole teacher of his work.

Over the years, the handful of apprentices who had studied with Pilates continued to develop his work, incorporate their own influences, and keep his method and approach to exercise alive. This first generation of teachers came from the New York City dance and theater community.

While Joseph Pilates was protective of his work, he never purchased any trademark for the term "Pilates." In fact, Pilates referred to his work as Contrology, a name that never became popular. He published two books, *Your Health* in 1934 and *Return to Life Through Contrology* in 1945. His second book, which he co-authored with William John Miller, contains pictures and descriptions of the 34 classical Pilates mat exercises. At first glance, a number of these exercises are physically reminiscent of classical hatha yoga poses and others appear to be modifications of yoga-inspired postures. In his original texts, however, Pilates does not mention from whom he learned yoga or mention the yogic tradition as an influence on his work. Moreover, unlike yoga, Pilates' complete system of exercise uses a variety of machines and aims to achieve physical and mental conditioning, not spiritual discovery. The practice of Pilates is not spiritual and does not incorporate the East Asian concept of life energy, also known as prana, chi, or ki, that is seen in yoga and certain martial arts.

In 1991, Joan Breibart initiated one of the earliest efforts to organize Pilates practitioners in the United States. She and Michele Larsson founded the Institute for the Pilates Method in Santa Fe, New Mexico, in consultation with Eve Gentry, one of Pilates' original apprentices. That same year, the Institute initiated the creation of the first national

Pilates teacher training and certification program, which continues to this day.

Through the leadership of early enthusiasts, the practice of Pilates exercise continued to grow and flourish in different parts of the world. The original Pilates Studio, however, was having consistent financial problems. Different individuals undertook efforts to finance continued operation of the Studio, including the filing of a Pilates trademark in 1980. Through various transfers, this trademark came into the possession of Sean Gallagher, a New York City–based physical therapist, who decided to try to enforce it. Beginning in 1992, he started threatening teachers and studios with legal action if they used the term Pilates to describe their businesses. Many practitioners and businesses— including the Institute for the Pilates Method, which became the Physicalmind Institute— changed the names of their organizations as a result of these legal threats to avoid any further legal entanglement.

In 1996, when Sean Gallagher filed suit against Balanced Body, an equipment manufacturer, and its owner Ken Endelman for trademark infringement, Endelman decided to challenge him. On October 20, 2000, a District Court judge in the Southern District of New York issued a decision that the term "Pilates" is generic both in reference to certain types of equipment and to exercise instruction services. As a practical matter, this decision meant that others are free to use the term Pilates to describe

those specific applications. In other words, no individual or business organization can claim exclusive ownership of the term Pilates to describe the style of exercise they teach or the equipment they manufacture. After this ruling a number of teachers, education providers, and equipment manufacturers changed the names of their businesses to include the term Pilates.

In 2001, the Pilates Method Alliance (PMA) was founded by Kevin A. Bowen and Colleen Glenn as a non-profit, unbiased information resource dedicated to the teachings of Joseph H. and Clara Pilates. Unlike other organizations that offer instructor training and certification programs, the PMA is a separate body with an organizational mission to protect the public by establishing certification and continuing education standards for Pilates professionals. One of the goals of the PMA is to create a national certification test for the Pilates method.

Growth

Today, variations of the Pilates method are practiced around the globe. According to the Superstudy® of Sports Participation by American Sports Data Inc., an estimated 4.7 million Americans practiced Pilates in 2003, an increase of more than 100% from the previous year, and most participants are females aged 38 and older. Participation is expected to increase due to consumer appeal, particularly among the growing number of aging baby boomers, and mounting medical evidence that mind-body exercise promotes overall health.

The many variations of Pilates are united by their common foundation and adherence to the basic principles of Pilates, which are covered in Chapter Two. Due to the similarity of Pilates to yoga, fusion-styled classes that blend Pilates exercises with hatha yoga postures are becoming increasingly popular. While these two disciplines are distinct, both yoga and Pilates have much to offer consumers on both a physical and mental level, because they not only offer physical conditioning benefits, but also require mental concentration that enhances the mind-body connection.

Benefits and Risks

The regular practice of Pilates mat exercise offers the following benefits for apparently healthy participants, in addition to improvements in overall strength, flexibility, stability, and mobility.

- improved posture
- stronger abdominal and back muscles
- stronger pelvic and shoulder stabilizer muscles
- balanced muscle development
- improved breathing
- better coordination and balance
- reduced likelihood of back pain or injury
- enhanced confidence and self-esteem
- enhanced mind-body connection
- enhanced athletic performance

Practicing Pilates provides these benefits because the exercises combine the use of the core musculature to stabilize the torso with rhythmic, coordinated movements accompanied by deep breathing. Precise attention to detail and form creates a stronger core and more efficient movement habits. This translates into better posture and more effective movement mechanics in both functional activities and in sports. In addition, imbalances in muscular development immediately become apparent and can be corrected by performing the exercises regularly and by progressing the level of difficulty over time.

With Pilates mat exercises, as with any exercise program, there is always a risk of injury. For this reason, it is important that fitness professionals ensure that adequate pre-screening has been conducted in accordance with industry standards and guidelines and that medical clearances are obtained as necessary. Check your *ACE Personal Trainer Manual* or *ACE Group Fitness Instructor Manual* for sample forms. In particular, because Pilates mat exercises involve spinal flexion, rotation, and extension, there is a higher risk of injury for individuals with orthopedic problems. In addition, certain Pilates exercises include high-risk hatha yoga poses such as the plow and the shoulderstand that should not be taught unless the instructor is highly experienced and trained, and the participants are ready and individually supervised.

Although Pilates is widely accepted in rehabilitation, trainers should not provide any training services beyond the appropriate scope of practice as defined by their specific training, certification, or licensure. As with all forms of exercise, fitness professionals should always consider the safety of the participant first, and only offer instructional services that are based on solid and in-depth training. Fitness professionals should not teach any movements without a complete understanding of the benefits and risks and of the necessary modifications for people with different body types and needs.

Pilates' Exercise Inventions

Joseph Pilates invented several apparatuses to complement his exercises. While none of these machines are featured in the exercises in this book, you will inevitably get some questions from participants regarding the use and benefits of some of his more widely used inventions.

Reformer—Inspired by a hospital bed, the reformer features a carriage that slides on top of a large rectangular frame. At one end of the frame is a foot bar. Two straps can be placed on the feet or hands for exercise variations. The exerciser works in a lying, standing, seated, kneeling, or lunging position. Springs that attach the carriage to the frame provide resistance (Figure 1.1).

Trapeze or Trap Table—Pilates created the inspiration for the trapeze table while imprisoned in a British internment camp, where he attached bed springs to walls above hospital beds to provide patients with a means to exercise while bedridden. This apparatus resembles a four-poster bed. At one end, approximately mid-way up the posts, is a spring-loaded "push through bar." At the other end are a variety of springs and a hanging bar that looks like a trapeze (Figure 1.2).

Wunda Chair—Pilates intended this exercise tool to double as a seat when not in use. It resembles a step stool with a padded seat and a movable foot bar. The foot bar is attached inside the frame of the stool with springs. Exercises are performed on the Wunda Chair by pushing the spring-loaded bar down and controlling the movement up with either the feet or the hands. Poles can be added to the sides to provide arm support for exercises performed when standing on top of the chair (Figure 1.3).

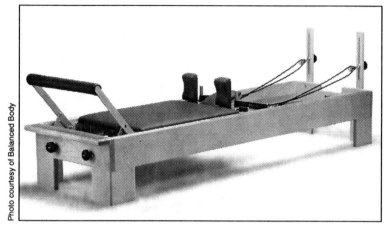

Figure 1.1
Reformer

Photo courtesy of Balanced Body

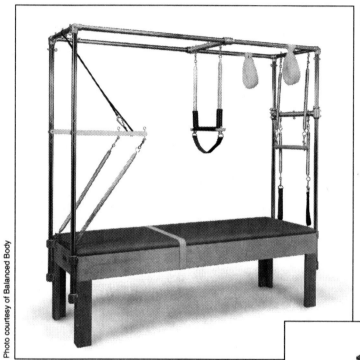

Figure 1.2
Trapeze Table

Photo courtesy of Balanced Body

Figure 1.3
Wunda Chair

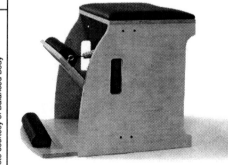

Photo courtesy of Balanced Body

The Six Traditional Pilates Principles

The purpose of Pilates training is to uniformly develop the body and the mind through a specific approach to exercise. This chapter describes the six Pilates principles and their application to the exercises to demonstrate why the Pilates method is unique from other styles of movement. Joseph Pilates drew on yoga, boxing, and even Chinese acrobatics, among other movement styles, to develop his training system. What makes Pilates distinct from those influences is the manner in which it incorporates the following six principles:

- Concentration
- Control
- Physical centering
- Flowing movement
- Precision
- Breathing

Every Pilates exercise should reflect these six principles when performed. Examined individually, none of these concepts is original in its application to movement disciplines. However, when systematically combined in the Pilates method, they form the unique quality that characterizes the practice of Pilates.

Concentration

Concentration is the first Pilates principle. Pilates encouraged developing mental power over the body in his writings. "One of the major results of Contrology [Pilates] is gaining the mastery of your mind over the complete control of your body" (Pilates & Miller, 1945). He emphasized the importance of paying attention to every movement, similar to the mental discipline required of the practice of yoga and East Asian martial arts. This link is an important connection between Pilates, a modern mind-body discipline, and the ancient mind-body disciplines of traditional East Asian cultures. The distinction in Pilates, however, is that it does not integrate this mind-body connection with the concept of life energy or universal energy. Instead, Pilates focused on the individual and believed that performing exercise while concentrating on the body was healthy for the brain and the body. He quoted G. Stanley Hall, an American psychologist who observed, "The culture of muscles is brain-building" (Pilates & Miller, 1945).

Correct execution of Pilates exercises demands concentration because they involve highly specific movement patterns requiring correct placement of every part of the body. This concentration leads to heightened body awareness. The Side Kick basic mat exercise illustrates the principle of concentration because you need to focus on stabilizing the pelvis, spine, and shoulder girdle to perform the movement correctly (see page 45). Some clients will enjoy this direct integration of the mind with the body while performing exercises. Those who prefer to exercise and focus more on background music, atmosphere, or other external stimuli are less likely to gravitate toward this style of concentrated exercise.

For exercisers who enjoy this type of mental engagement with their movement activities, however, Pilates can be a perfect fit. With practice, concentrating on micro-movements becomes easier and translates into an improved mind-body connection that results in greater body awareness both on and off the training mat.

Research in exercise science supports the observation that concentrating on movement activities is healthy for the brain and suggests that regular physical activity, because it stimulates the brain and the neuromuscular system to perform coordinated patterns, helps to prevent or deter the onset of diseases that impair cognitive faculties in older adults (American Council on Exercise, 1998). Exercise is as important to the health of the mind as it is to the body—providing more evidence to support the strong connection between the two. Health of body and health of mind must co-exist and support each other.

Control

Pilates, which was initially called Contrology, was founded on the principle of control. "Contrology [Pilates] begins with mind control over the body" (Pilates & Miller, 1945). This emphasis on control is one of the reasons why Pilates did not recommend performing a high number of repetitions of each exercise. He believed that a few repetitions, executed with control and concentration, provide the best training. In *Return to Life Through Contrology,* Pilates writes, "Concentrate on the correct movements EACH TIME YOU EXERCISE, lest you do them improperly and thus lose all the vital benefits of their value. Correctly executed and mastered to the point of subconscious reaction, these exercises will reflect grace and balance in your routine activities" (Pilates & Miller, 1945).

The exercise Rolling Back exemplifies this principle (see page 48). By using coordinated breathing patterns and activation of deep abdominal muscles, the exerciser can control the rolling of the body on the spine. If the exerciser loses control while rolling, the mind-body connection with the essential deep abdominal muscles is lost. In other words, the participant cannot succeed at this exercise without

exercising control over the body and making the mind-body connection.

Applying the principle of control during exercise provides many benefits. Primarily, it serves to improve the mind-body connection of the practitioner. In addition, a controlled approach to training builds better body awareness, reduces the likelihood of injury, and improves neuromuscular development.

Physical Centering

Centering, or strengthening the body's physical center, is a focal point of the Pilates method of exercise. A stronger and more toned "powerhouse," a term commonly used by Pilates instructors to describe the body's center, is one of the primary results of Pilates training. The powerhouse refers to the torso area between the bottom of the rib cage and the top of the pelvis or ilium. In Pilates, this "center" is purely a physical center, not a spiritual one as in many East Asian movement arts. The muscles in this part of the body support the spine, internal organs, and posture. Most Pilates exercises require you to stabilize the body's physical center before executing additional arm, leg, and torso movements. This is also sometimes referred to as "training from the inside out," because as the body's deep intrinsic muscles begin to activate and perform their intended supportive functions, more superficial "global" muscles become more efficient. All of the muscles can begin to work more synergistically and efficiently, each performing its intended function.

The principle of centering is consistent with Pilates' belief in the importance of good posture. "The art of Contrology [Pilates] proves that the only real guide to your true age lies not in years or how you think you feel, but as you actually are, as infallibly indicated by the degree of natural and normal flexibility enjoyed by your spine throughout life" (Pilates & Miller, 1945).

The principle of centering is applied in every Pilates exercise. The Leg Slides exercise exemplifies this principle (see page 32). In this exercise, the body is stabilized in a supine position as the heels alternately slide away from the pelvis until the leg is extended as far as possible without moving the pelvis. Leg Slides are impossible to perform without strong core muscles to maintain neutral spinal alignment throughout the exercise. All of the body's muscles, both intrinsic and superficial, must optimally perform their intended functions to create both stability and mobility for precise and flowing execution of the exercise.

In our modern culture, most people will benefit from conditioning exercises that target the body's center. Up to 80% of American adults will experience back pain at some point in their adult life, and back pain is the leading cause of absence from work. Most individuals also experience neck and shoulder tension. At the same time, a strong physical center is essential for optimizing physical performance. This principle, therefore, has something to offer every exerciser, from beginner to athlete.

Flowing Movement

The next Pilates principle is flowing movement. Ideally, the practitioner should execute Pilates exercises in a fluid, natural manner without jerky starts and sudden stops. "Through Contrology [Pilates] you first purposefully acquire complete control of your own body and then through proper repetition of its exercises you gradually acquire rhythm and coordination associated with all your subconscious activities" (Pilates & Miller, 1945). This principle is complementary to the principles of concentration, control, and precision. After the exerciser focuses the mind on the body, he or she must then learn to release excess tension so movements are smooth and flow evenly.

The Modified Swan Dive is one of many Pilates exercises that exemplify this principle of flowing movement or grace (see page 56). The Modified Swan Dive, which requires both strength and flexibility, is performed in a continuous pattern with each repetition blending seamlessly into the next. While coordinating breathing with motion, the practitioner rolls forward and back from a prone position with spinal and hip extension.

This aspect of Pilates practice is likely to have been influenced by traditional East Asian disciplines, as they all incorporate the concept of fluid, flowing motion. Tai chi chuan is a form of slow, meditative shadowboxing. Fluid, controlled movement also characterizes the ancient arts of qigong and yoga, both of which cultivate strength, flexibility, and balance, and feature moving limbs in imitation of the stances of animals in nature. Pilates was also fascinated by and studied the movement patterns of animals.

Precision

Pilates believed that precise attention to subtle movement details helped to train the body and mind to move more efficiently at all times. Therefore, precise execution of every aspect of each exercise is vital to this discipline, and can result in balanced muscle development and smooth, efficient movement.

Contemporary research in the mind-body relationship supports the concept that focused attention of the mind enhances training and that the most efficient training results from focusing on proper execution (LaForge, 2003). For example, to learn a new sports skill such as golf or tennis, pros advise newcomers to learn proper form from the beginning, to practice correct execution, and to stop practicing when mentally unable to focus on good form. This approach to training is embodied by the principle of precision.

Breathing

Finally, the principle of using the breath to enhance movement is essential to the authentic performance of Pilates exercises. Pilates was a strong believer in using the breath as a vehicle to energize the body. The exerciser should use full inhalations and exhalations with each repetition. "Squeeze out the lungs as you would ring a wet towel dry. Soon the entire body is charged with fresh oxygen from toes to fingertips, just as the head of steam in a boiler rushes to every radiator in the house" (Pilates & Miller, 1945). Each Pilates exercise has movement patterns that are coordinated with breathing patterns. Coordinating these patterns is a fundamental feature of Pilates exercises.

This principle is also consistent with traditional mind-body disciplines such as yoga, tai chi, and East Asian martial arts that all strongly feature attention to breathing and the coordination of breath with movement. By focusing on breath, the practitioner is immediately brought into what is called present-state awareness, in which the mind cannot wander to worry about other topics, but instead must engage in a singular connection with the body in the moment. This is an essential feature of all mind-body disciplines.

Modern Concepts

Pilates passed away in 1967, but his work endures. As each generation of teachers continues to teach his principles, Pilates training has evolved and remained vital through the incorporation of additional concepts. Examples of recent additions to the Pilates system that reflect perspectives from physical therapy and modern exercise science include towel work and the use of percussive breathing with exercises; the concept of "imprinting" the spine; the use of Pilates in sports medicine and rehabilitation; and an emphasis placed on neutral alignment.

These concepts and techniques provide a modern evolving edge that adds value to Pilates for today's consumer. Some purists believe that if the exercises are not presented exactly in the same way that Joseph Pilates taught them, then it is not Pilates. Other experts believe that if the exercises remain true to the original principles and spirit of the work, then it is still Pilates. It is a testament to the strength of Joseph Pilates' original work that his system of exercises has stood the test of time and evolved with modern influences. Fitness professionals should be mindful of the classical Pilates principles and understand the conceptual framework and spirit within which the exercises were originally taught.

At the same time, fitness professionals must continually update their knowledge and adapt movements in accordance with new, accepted industry standards to ensure that all forms of conditioning exercises, including Pilates mat exercises, are taught safely and effectively. There are multiple levels of competency in teaching and fitness instructors should only teach the exercises for which they have received professional training. Fitness professionals who want to become teachers of Pilates will need to pursue professional training that adheres to the principles of Pilates and also incorporates contemporary knowledge of exercise science and biomechanics.

Modern Exercise Science

CHAPTER THREE

The purpose of this chapter is to examine the Pilates exercise system from the perspective of modern exercise science and offer a deeper understanding of the purpose and benefits of Pilates training. Joseph Pilates developed his method based on his own experience and understanding of the body through his own training, from what he learned from others in multiple movement disciplines, and by training his own clients. He also spent countless hours observing movement patterns of animals and infants, similar to the practices of ancient East Asian martial artists and yogis. Many of his exercises appear to draw inspiration from traditional hatha yoga postures. He did not have an exercise science degree, nor did he approach the work from that perspective. This contemporary analysis, therefore, is not from the point of view of how the exercises were originally created.

Joseph Pilates passionately believed in the importance of good posture and a healthy spine. To achieve those ends, he designed mat and equipment exercises to improve the postural and movement habits of his clients with a focus on conditioning the muscles in the body's center, both to recover from injury and to prevent future injuries. Today, this category of exercises typically is described as core stabilization. Keep in mind, however, that Pilates did not design his exercises with the concept of core stabilization in mind, but rather developed exercise programs to improve the posture and movement of his specific clientele, considering the need for stability and mobility for efficient movement.

To progress clients to more difficult levels of challenge, mat exercises incorporate limb movements with varying ranges of motion, lever lengths, and bases of support. In contrast, equipment-based exercises allow for modifications by providing both assistance and resistance to limb movements. Throughout the exercise design, the roles of stability and mobility continue to be emphasized and challenged.

Within the Pilates community, some practitioners believe that the exercises should be taught in exactly the same way that Joseph and Clara Pilates taught them 70 years ago. Some of these practitioners adopt what can be described as a choreographic approach with sequencing and positions that do not lend themselves to modifications for individual students. This approach is not recommended, because standards of professional responsibility require that exercise be both safe and effective for the individual exerciser.

Modern applications of the Pilates method incorporate what we have learned from the study of biomechanics and how the physical laws of motion govern movement of the human body, as well as what we have learned from the fields of exercise science and physical therapy. This approach yields what are sometimes referred to as "evolved," "contemporary," "inspired," or "re-invented" versions of Pilates.

Because this book is intended for certified fitness professionals, it will approach the practice of Pilates as a fitness activity that can meet safety and quality objectives to promote the benefits of physical activity for all segments of society. This chapter examines the primary exercise science concepts and training principles that are applied to Pilates.

As the fitness industry continues to evolve to meet consumer needs, the field of exercise science and biomechanics continues to explore human movement science. The trend toward functional training has emerged with an aim of improving conditioning strategies. Addressing separate aspects of fitness, such as cardio-vascular training, muscle conditioning, flexibility training, and balance and coordination training, is essential in a well-balanced training program. However, it is also important to consider how the body moves as an integrated functional unit. An integrated approach incorporates training the muscular, nervous, and skeletal systems. Good posture or ideal alignment affects the body's ability to move. To train effectively, you must have an understanding of postural deviations and the important role of good posture.

Common Postural Deviations

Most people do not possess ideal postural alignment. Common postural deviations include kyphosis-lordosis, the flat-back posture, and the sway-back posture. These conditions contribute to inflammation, chronic pain, and injury.

Kyphosis-lordosis

Kyphosis-lordosis is an increase in the normal inward curve of the low back, often accompanied by a protruding abdomen and buttocks (lordosis), increased flexion (outward curve) of the thoracic spine, rounded shoulders, and a forward-tilted head (kyphosis) (Figure 3.1). The person with this posture typically has tight lower-back muscles, hip flexors, internal obliques, shoulder adductors, and intercostals. Weak muscles include the abdominals (especially obliques), hip extensors, erector spinae of the thoracic spine, and scapular adductors.

Flat-back

Flat-back posture is a decrease in the normal inward curve of the lower back, with the pelvis in posterior tilt (Figure 3.2). The person with this posture often has tight upper abdominals and hip extensors, and the body appears rigid. Weak muscles include those of the lower back and the hip flexors.

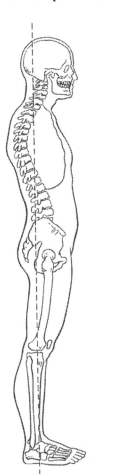

Figure 3.1
Kyphosis-lordosis posture

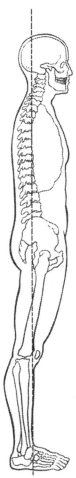

Figure 3.2
Flat-back posture

Sway-back

The sway-back posture is a long outward curve of the thoracic spine with an accentuated lumbar curve and a backward shift of the upper trunk (Figure 3.3). It is often accompanied by rounded shoulders, a sunken chest, and a forward-tilted head. The person with this posture usually has tight upper abdominals and hip flexors. Weak muscles include oblique abdominals and hip extensors.

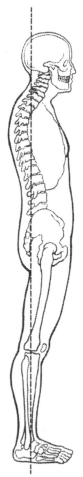

Figure 3.3
Sway-back posture

Neutral Alignment

Neutral alignment promotes ideal functional movement. Good posture maintains structural integrity, enables the development of functional strength and neuromuscular efficiency, and reduces the likelihood of joint strain and injury. In addition to the conditioning benefits to the abdominal and back muscles, one of the greatest physical benefits of regular Pilates practice is improved posture and enhanced movement efficiency.

Neutral Alignment and the Pilates Method

Leading teachers of the Pilates method today continue to develop or "evolve" the system of exercises to incorporate contemporary knowledge and to meet the changing needs of clients. While it is true that Pilates believed that a healthy spine was a flat spine, his belief must be understood in the historical context of when he was working. In the 1920s, Pilates did not have access to today's modern technology, nor to the research we now have regarding spinal biomechanics. Furthermore, the clientele that he was working with in New York, who were primarily professional dancers with a highly developed sense of body awareness, did not have the same needs as the majority of today's typical exercisers. In addition, even among clients who were not dancers or athletes, previous generations enjoyed a more active lifestyle than Americans today. Fitness professionals are now called upon to work with individuals who may have very little body awareness and may be leading extremely sedentary lifestyles.

Eve Gentry is credited with first moving away from the flat-back position through her technique of "imprinting," which involves releasing tension from the muscles along the spine while lying in a supine position without pressing the lower back into the mat. This emphasis on training in neutral spine has been further developed by many Pilates educators who advocate the integration of modern exercise science into the traditional teachings of Pilates.

The teaching of contemporary Pilates emphasizes training from the inside out, and trains these intrinsic muscles to stabilize a neutral postural alignment and to create an efficient gait pattern. The spine is in neutral alignment when the ear, shoulder, hip, knee, and ankle line up with each other along a vertical plumb line. The natural "S" shape of the spinal column is retained. The discs are not compressed, nor are any of the spinal curves hyperextended (Figure 3.4). Maintaining neutral spinal alignment helps to avoid back pain and injuries, and the compression of nerves that run through the spinal column. For athletes, conditioning muscles that stabilize neutral alignment facilitates more efficient transfer of forces through the limbs, resulting in greater speed and power.

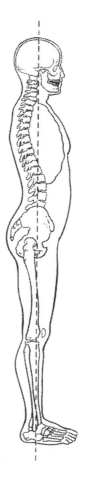

Figure 3.4
Ideal (neutral) alignment

Core Stabilization

For athletic coaches, core stabilization training generally targets the muscles of the lumbo-pelvic-hip complex to improve dynamic postural control. For the purposes of Pilates, however, core stabilization is expanded to include trunk and shoulder stabilization and lumbopelvic control. This expanded vision of the core can produce more efficient movement patterns. Pilates exercises re-train the neuromuscular system while conditioning the body by putting the exerciser through dynamic coordinated movements that require the exerciser to stabilize the entire torso. This training approach helps to create new movement habits that result in more balanced muscles, greater comfort, and physical control. Examining each of these specific areas provides a clearer picture of some of the physiological foundations of this system of exercise.

Trunk Stabilizers

The Pilates system begins by targeting the muscles in the body's center, or the trunk stabilizers, which include both the abdominal and back muscle groups working together to support the spine. The abdominal muscle group exists in four layers, each of which serves a different purpose. These deep muscles of the spine connect each of the 25 vertebrae to its adjacent vertebrae and span the entire length of the spinal column. Based on available evidence, scientists believe that the deepest muscles provide important "position sense" information to the brain regarding where the vertebrae are in space and also increase stiffness within the spinal structure itself (Bogduk, 1997; Crisco & Panjabi, 1991). This position sense information is critical to our sense of balance, which of course enhances stability as it dictates the degree of stiffness of the spine.

Researchers believe that the middle layer of trunk musculature provides the most essential muscular "bracing" of the spine, particularly to the lower back. These middle-layer muscles include back muscles (multifidus and quadratus lumborum) and abdominal muscles (the transverse abdominis and internal obliques), and support the spinal column in various positions and help to prevent injuries. Athletes, in particular, need strong spinal stabilizers to improve the transfer of forces to the arms and legs for greater movement control and increased speed and power.

Interestingly, researchers have determined that the multifidi have six times more muscle spindles than any other muscle in the trunk. It is theorized, therefore, that these muscles also play an important role in movement control and position sense awareness, or proprioception. Researchers have noted that in people with low-back pain, the multifidi muscles are not typically working at optimal functional ability (Bogduk, 1997; Crisco & Panjabi, 1991; Clark, 2001). Because modern Pilates exercises require maintenance of neutral spinal alignment at varying levels of challenge, these muscles can be conditioned, thus improving posture and functional mobility. This is not to suggest that Pilates instructors should assume a role as a clinical rehabilitation specialist for people with special needs. Rather, the practice of Pilates exercises may offer valuable conditioning that could possibly prevent low-back pain in those who have not yet developed the condition.

Some scientists believe that the transverse abdominis is the primary muscle in postural control and provides torso support much like a girdle (Hodges & Richardson, 1996). The

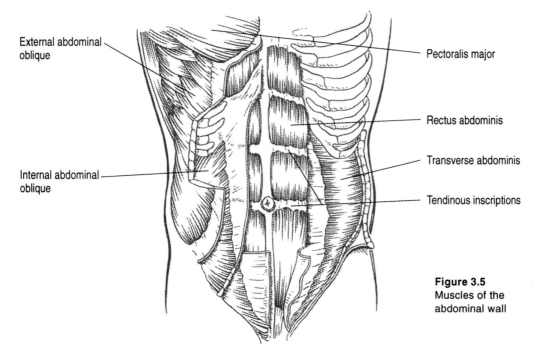

External abdominal oblique

Internal abdominal oblique

Pectoralis major

Rectus abdominis

Transverse abdominis

Tendinous inscriptions

Figure 3.5
Muscles of the abdominal wall

transverse abdominis works best at a submaximal contraction and is optimally trained when the spine is in neutral alignment, as its fibers run horizontally and it encircles the abdominal cavity (Figure 3.5). Other researchers believe that no single muscle possesses a dominant role in spinal stability, but rather that stabilization results from a number of muscles working together synergistically (Cholewicki & McGill, 1996; Cholewicki & Van Vliet, 2002).

The outermost layer of trunk muscles moves the torso in flexion, extension, and rotation using the following muscles: the erector spinae in the back, and the external obliques and rectus abdominis along the sides and front. In contrast to the stabilizers, these muscles function more as prime mover muscles, while some scientists believe that these more superficial muscles also play a role in stabilization. In Pilates exercises,

the focus is on ensuring activation of both the deeper stabilizer muscles as well as these prime movers. Therefore, in exercises such as The Hundred I or II (see pages 46–47), the emphasis is placed first on the stabilizers—then the difficulty progressed only as the stabilizers can handle the increase in workload—rather than adjusted to meet the strength of the usually stronger rectus abdominis. According to students of Joseph Pilates, he emphasized stabilizing the body from the powerhouse first, before initiating movement, which is the ideal approach to condition stabilizer muscles. In this manner, practitioners can benefit from "training from the inside out."

Available research shows that the most effective training for the trunk is balanced in its approach and targets each muscular layer to optimize spinal stabilization and overall fitness.

Studies show that the relative contribution of muscles to spinal stability varies depending on the forces involved (Kavcic, Grenier, & McGill, 2004). Therefore, some suggest that optimal training may result from enhancing motor patterns that incorporate many muscles, rather than targeting each individual muscle with separate exercises. Joseph Pilates referred to use of these deeper muscles as the principle of "centering." East Asian movement disciplines have referred to training from the body's center, known as the t'an tien or hara, for thousands of years.

Shoulder Girdle Stabilizers

In addition to trunk stabilization, Pilates exercises also focus on shoulder girdle stabilization as it relates to neutral alignment and core stabilization. The shoulder girdle stabilizer muscles include the trapezius, rhomboids, levator scapulae, serratus anterior, and pectoralis minor (Figures 3.6 & 3.7). The primary role of the shoulder girdle stabilizers is to maintain optimal function and alignment of the shoulder joint and the scapulae with respect to the thoracic spine. If any muscular imbalances are present, the integrity of the shoulder joint is compromised. By challenging the shoulder girdle muscles to work effectively under varying loads and in different ranges of motion, the Pilates approach conditions the muscles that surround the joint to improve efficiency and reduce the likelihood of injury.

The serratus anterior connects to the upper eight or nine ribs and to the entire medial border of the scapula. The serratus anterior holds the scapula against the ribs and functions to protract

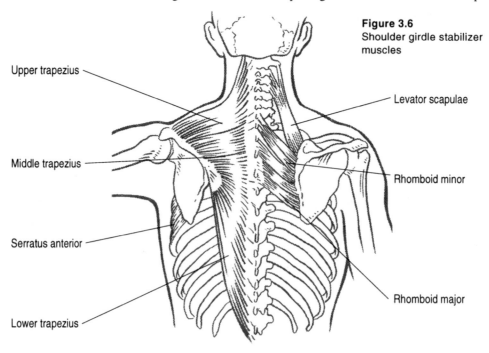

Figure 3.6
Shoulder girdle stabilizer muscles

Upper trapezius

Levator scapulae

Middle trapezius

Rhomboid minor

Serratus anterior

Rhomboid major

Lower trapezius

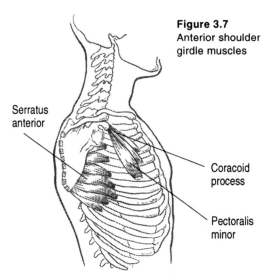

Figure 3.7
Anterior shoulder girdle muscles

Serratus anterior

Coracoid process

Pectoralis minor

spinous processes and the medial border of the scapula. The rhomboids work to retract and elevate the scapula. Like the middle trapezius, the rhomboids are often weak in people with a sedentary lifestyle.

The trapezius is the largest and most super-ficial shoulder girdle–muscle stabilizer. The functions of the trapezius include scapular elevation, depression, retraction, and upward rotation, and the upper trapezius facilitates head and neck extension, lateral flexion, and rotation to the opposite side. The trapezius functions at an optimal level when the upper, middle, and lower regions are in balance. The lower trapezius plays an important role in dynamic scapular stabi-lization. With our contemporary seated lifestyle, many people typically have short, tight upper-trapezius muscles and weak, over-stretched middle- and lower-trapezius muscles. Targeted training can improve muscular balance and reduce the likelihood of injury or chronic pain.

Muscular imbalances among these shoulder girdle stabilizers adversely affect posture and can result in rounded shoulders and a collapsed chest. Over time, this postural pattern can lead to rotator cuff impingement, shoulder instability, and headaches, among other injuries. Using proper posture when training, as is emphasized throughout contemporary Pilates training, is among the most effective methods to begin correcting this condition.

and upwardly rotate the scapula. It works together with the middle trapezius to stabilize the scapula and, together with the lower trapezius, to rotate the scapula upward and outward.

The pectoralis minor connects to ribs three to five and inserts on the coracoid process. The pectoralis minor depresses the scapula and moves it forward and down. If it is tight and short, it can overly pull the scapula forward. It also assists in respiration by elevating the ribs upon inspiration.

The levator scapulae connect the superior medial area of the scapula to the cervical vertebrae and lie beneath the upper trapezius. The function of the levator scapulae is scapular elevation and downward and inward rotation. In most individuals, these muscles are short and tight.

The rhomboids are deeper than the trapezius and lie beneath the middle and upper trapezius and in between the scapula. They connect to the

Pelvic Stabilizers

Conditioning the pelvic stabilizers is another key element of the Pilates method. Due to the close relationship of the pelvis and the lumbar spine, the pelvic stabilizer muscles include the deep abdominal and back muscles that co-contract to maintain a neutral lumbar spine. A neutral pelvic position is present when a neutral lumbar spine position is present. Some exercise scientists also believe that the pelvic floor and diaphragm muscles play a stabilizing role.

In addition to achieving a stable position forward and back in the sagittal plane, the pelvis also ideally needs to be stabilized in the frontal and transverse planes. The external rotators and hip abductors function as both mover muscles and pelvic stabilizers. The external rotators prevent the pelvis from tilting laterally in the frontal plane to help maintain alignment. The hip abductors (gluteus medius and minimus and tensor fascia latae) also prevent lateral tilting and help stabilize the pelvis (ilium) around the hip joint. The hip adductors primarily stabilize the thighs and internally rotate the hips.

Neutral pelvis and neutral lumbar spine exist when the pelvis is in a central position and is neither flexed, extended, tilted, nor rotated. To understand the varieties of pelvic positioning, the pelvis may be compared to a bucket of water. If the bucket is tilted in any direction: front, back, or to either side, the water will spill (Figure 3.8). If a muscular imbalance is present,

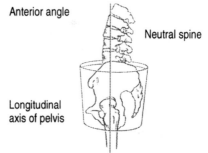

Neutral lumbar spine with neutral pelvis

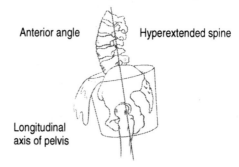

Lumbar hyperextension with anterior pelvic tilt

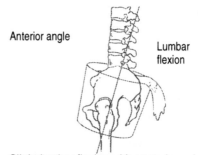

Slight lumbar flexion with posterior pelvic tilt

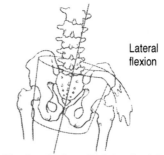

Lateral lumbar flexion with lateral pelvic tilt

Figure 3.8
Pelvic tilt can be anterior, posterior, or lateral. The bucket of water serves as a visual aid to better illustrate the direction of the pelvic tilt.

tighter hamstrings or hip flexors can pull the pelvis either too far back or too far forward, resulting in lower-back strain and loss of pelvic stability. Weak external rotators can allow the hip to rotate forward or tilt laterally. Weak hip abductors contribute to lateral tilting of the pelvis. These pelvic deviations can also lead to stress and injury in the hip joints.

Because the pelvis and lumbar spine are closely related, muscular imbalances that affect pelvic stability can also pull the lumbar spine out of its neutral position. For example, tight hamstrings can cause a posterior tilt or "flat-back" position and tight hip flexors can cause an anterior tilt or "sway-back" position. Any muscular imbalances around the pelvis, therefore, need to be addressed to support a stable neutral posture.

The Value of Pilates Training for Fitness Professionals

The Pilates method focuses on total-body training and balanced muscular development. Evidence from research in exercise science points to the importance of training clients in the positions required by activities of daily living and sport-specific training to include neutral spinal alignment, spine flexion, extension, rotation, lateral translation, and combined planes of motion to create optimal structural and functional efficiency. When deeper stabilizer muscles are weak, more superficial mover muscles must compensate for their inactivity. These muscles can then become tight, leading to chronic tension since they are not intended to play a bracing role. Over time, this muscular tightness causes reciprocal inhibition of muscle antagonists, further increasing muscular and structural weakness. The long-term result is compromised alignment, joint dysfunction, and neuromuscular inefficiency leading to pain and injury.

Current exercise guidelines recommend that participants engage in cardiovascular training, muscular conditioning, and flexibility training for health. Exercise scientists now recognize the importance of good postural alignment during physical activities. The incorporation of Pilates exercises into an exercise program therefore increases the likelihood that structural integrity will be present in other activities.

Fitness professionals need to understand the importance of good alignment when training. Since the Pilates method of exercise focuses on conditioning the body's stabilizer muscles, and contemporary Pilates includes stabilizing in neutral alignment, weak muscles can become stronger, tight muscles can be stretched, and proper movement patterns can be re-established. This forms a complementary basis for all movement training and can be a valuable addition to any client's overall exercise program with goals of improving conditioning, preventing injuries, and enhancing performance.

Basic

Mat

Exercises

CHAPTER FOUR

This chapter introduces a sampling of the foundation movements that can also be used as a warm-up, basic mat exercises, and suggestions for how to sequence exercises for balanced training and smooth teaching (page 62). Additional training in the Pilates method is recommended for a more comprehensive understanding of the complete system of exercises, which by some estimates includes as many as 500 exercises. Each exercise listed here is categorized as Beginner, Intermediate, or Advanced.

Foundation or Warm-up Exercises

1. Base Position (Supine Neutral Spine)
2. Pilates Breathing
3. Pelvic Tilt
4. Pelvic Clock
5. Bridge (Articulating Bridge)
6. Shoulder Slaps (Alternating Scapular Protraction and Neutral)
7. Rib Cage Arms (Supine Arm Arcs)
8. Leg Slides
9. Curl-up with Long Arms (Articulating Curl-up)
10. Chest Raise (Prone Cervical and Thoracic Extension)
11. Leg Lifts (Prone Hip Extension)
12. Knee Sways Stretch (Supine Spinal Rotation)
13. Knee Hug Stretch
14. Shell Stretch
15. Cat Stretch (Quadruped Spine Flexion)

Basic Mat Exercises

The following Pilates mat exercises have been organized according to type of movement: core stabilization, flexion, extension, or rotation. Some of the more difficult exercises have been broken down into a preparatory version and a standard version for stronger participants. Some exercises include variations and modifications to increase or decrease the level of intensity.

Core Stabilization

16. Modified Plank
17. Modified Scapular Push-up (Quadruped Scapular Push-up)
18. Upward Facing Leg Pull, Prep (Modified Supine Plank)
19. Side Bend Prep (Side Plank)

20. Side Bend
21. Side Kick

Flexion

22. The Hundred I
23. The Hundred II
24. Rolling Back
25. Single-leg Stretch
26. Spine Stretch (Seated Spine Flexion)

Extension

27. Swimming
28. Modified Swan Dive

Any exercise that involves spinal extension or flexion poses a risk of injury to participants who have any adverse spinal condition, particularly in the lumbar spine. Before teaching these exercises, always ensure that your participants have a healthy back and that they do not experience pain with any exercise.

Rotation

29. Spine Twist (Seated Spine Rotation)
30. Crisscross (Supine Single-leg Stretch with Trunk Rotation)

Foundation or Warm-up Exercises

The 15 exercises described here are all Beginner level movements. Joseph Pilates did not use these exercises in his original repertoire, with the exception of the Shell Stretch. These exercise are sometimes referred to as "pre-Pilates." They can be used as a complete workout for newcomers to Pilates or as a warm-up for more advanced exercisers.

1. Base Position (Supine Neutral Spine)

- Lie supine, with your knees flexed 90 degrees, feet flat on the mat, heels aligned with the ischium, and arms extended palms-down at your sides.
- Tilt your pelvis posteriorly until your lower back contacts the mat.
- Tilt your pelvis anteriorly until you are in a slightly arched-back position.
- Lie between these two extremes in a "neutral pelvis" position.
- Elevate your shoulders, then depress them. With your shoulders lowered, widen the scapulae and keep your rib cage in contact with the mat.

Maintain a neutral neck position. If the neck hyperextends, put a rolled towel or pillow under your head. This neutral spinal alignment is the Base Position (Figure 4.1).

If your back is not comfortable with the knees flexed 90 degrees, modify this position by sliding the heels farther away from the hips or by keeping one knee flexed and the other extended (Figure 4.2).

Note: Many Pilates and yoga instructors will use the descriptive term "sitz bones" when cueing in place of "ischium." Many of your participants or clients may be more familiar with this less technical terminology.

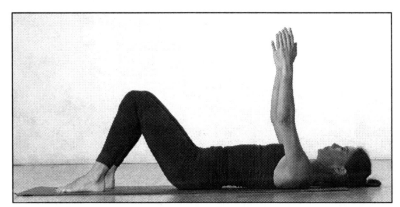

Note: Arms are elevated here to better show neutral spine. Arms are to be extended palms-down at your sides.

Figure 4.1
Base Position

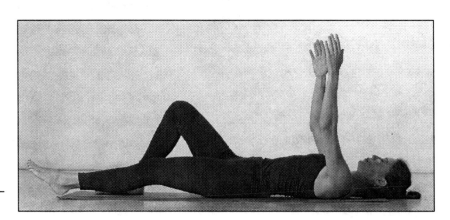

Figure 4.2
Base Position—
modification

2. Pilates Breathing

- Lie supine in the Base Position. Place your palms on the sides and top of your lower rib cage.
- Inhale and exhale naturally, observing any trunk movements.
- With your next exhalation, draw the pelvic floor upward.
- Inhale; feel the expansion of your torso with the breath.
- Exhale; draw the pelvic floor upward and contract the deep abdominals.
- Inhale; feel your torso expand wide and keep your rib cage connected with the mat.
- Exhale; activate your pelvic floor, deep abdominals, obliques, and intercostals as you feel the narrowing of the waist with the outflow of breath.
- With each inhalation, allow air to flow in. Contract your muscles while exhaling.

    Caution: Avoid excessive muscular effort when breathing. If you are new to breathing exercises, you may "over-breathe" and feel a sensation of dizziness from hyperventilation. Stop breathing exercises if you start to feel lightheaded. Simply breathe naturally. As you become used to deeper breathing, over-breathing should not be a problem.

3. Pelvic Tilt

- Lie supine in the Base Position with your arms extended palms-down at your sides.
- Inhale; remain in the neutral pelvis position, between a flat-back and an arched-back position.

- Exhaling, contract the deep abdominals. Feel your pelvis tilt gently and posteriorly without contracting the gluteal muscles and pushing the lower back into the mat. The posterior pelvic tilt should be experienced as a decompressive, elongating movement.
- Inhaling, return to neutral pelvis; lengthen the waist.
- This movement is subtle. Try to use abdominal muscles and not the strong muscles of your buttocks to draw the lower back toward the mat.

    This movement is often described as "imprinting" the spine, a term coined by Eve Gentry. She equated it with the sensation of lying in sand on a beach where you can allow the spine to relax, releasing any sense of compression among the individual vertebrae.

4. Pelvic Clock

- Lie supine in the Base Position with your arms extended palms-down at your sides.
- Imagine a clock face on your lower back: twelve o'clock is behind your navel; three o'clock is behind your left hip; six o'clock is the tip of your tailbone; nine o'clock is behind your right hip (Figure 4.3).
- Inhale as you press your tailbone into the mat at six o'clock (anterior pelvic tilt). Exhale as you press each hour of the clock in a clockwise motion against the mat (with twelve o'clock being a posterior pelvic tilt). Keep your feet, knees, and legs as still as possible. Feel the movement of your spine and pelvis as well as your abdominal and back muscles.

Moshe Feldenkrais created the "Pelvic Clock" exercise for use in his "Awareness Through Movement" lessons. Joseph Pilates did not use this exercise in his original repertoire. Leading Pilates educators integrated the "Pelvic Clock" into the warm-up routines that were created to supplement Pilates' original work.

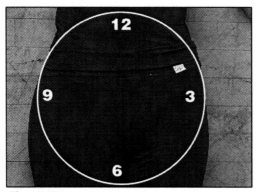

Figure 4.3
Pelvic Clock

5. Bridge (Articulating Bridge)

- Lie supine in the Base Position with your arms extended at your sides.

- Move your heels closer to your hips and depress the scapulae. Exhaling, slowly tilt the pelvis, lifting the lower back off the mat.

- Continue lifting your spine off the mat, one vertebra at a time, stopping when you reach the shoulders. Inhale and hold this position; rest on the shoulders and feet (Figure 4.4).

- Exhaling, slowly roll down, one vertebra at a time, to the Base Position.

Variation:

- To increase intensity, add Rib Cage Arm movements in the elevated bridge position by raising and then lowering your arms in an arc (Figure 4.5). Return your arms down to the sides before lowering back to the Base Position.

Caution: Stop if you have any lower-back pain or discomfort. Instead, perform the Pelvic Tilt until your strength increases (see page 28). Perform Knee Hug Stretch to release any tension from the lower back (see page 37).

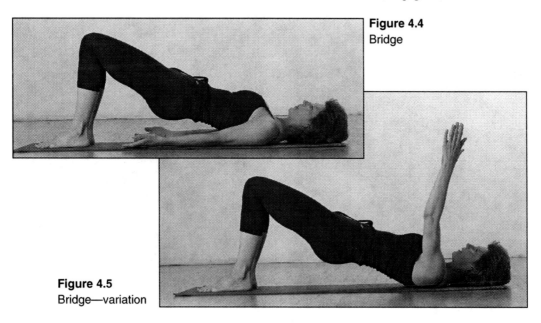

Figure 4.4
Bridge

Figure 4.5
Bridge—variation

6. Shoulder Slaps (Alternating Scapular Protraction and Neutral)

• Lie supine in the Base Position with your arms extended palms-down at your sides.

• Inhaling, lift both arms straight up above your shoulders, rotating the palms toward each other.

• Exhale and drop your scapulae to the mat (Figure 4.6a).

• Breathing naturally, lift one arm and then the other upward by lifting and dropping the scapulae, gently "slapping" the scapulae against the mat (Figure 4.6b).

• Stretch between the scapulae in the upper-middle back by reaching both hands toward the ceiling (Figure 4.6c).

• To finish, soften your chest, then inhale. Exhaling, bring your arms down to your sides to the Base Position.

Figure 4.6
Shoulder Slaps

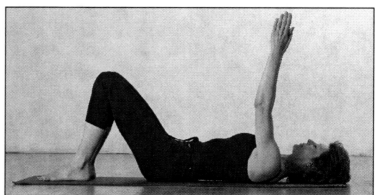

a.

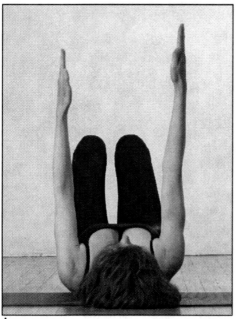

b.

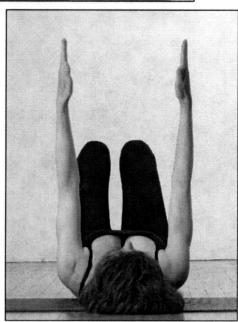

c.

7. Rib Cage Arms (Supine Arm Arcs)

• Lie on your back in the Base Position with your arms extended palms-down at your sides.

• Inhaling, lift both arms straight up above the shoulders, rotating your palms toward each other.

• Exhaling, continue the arcing motion overhead, extending your arms past your ears in a gentle V shape. Stabilize your shoulders. Keep your rib cage down; only arc your arms as far as possible without lifting your ribs off the mat. Maintain neutral spinal alignment while stretching the chest and anterior shoulders (Figure 4.7a).

• Inhaling, arc your arms upward, palms in. Keep your rib cage against the mat (Figure 4.7b).

• Exhaling, continue to arc your arms back down to the sides, palms down, returning to the Base Position.

Caution: Move within a comfortable range of motion and maintain neutral spine curves. Stop if you have any neck or shoulder pain or discomfort.

Figure 4.7
Rib Cage Arms

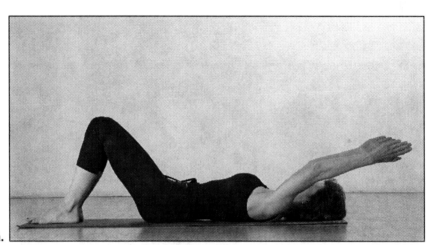

a.

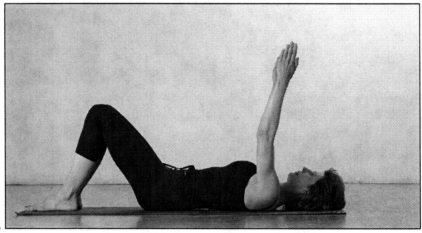

b.

8. Leg Slides

- Lie supine in the Base Position with your arms extended palms-down at your sides.
- Inhale to prepare.
- Exhaling, extend one leg by sliding the heel away from the pelvis. Only slide the heel as far as possible without moving the pelvis. Avoid a flat-back or an arched-back position and maintain neutral spinal alignment (Figure 4.8).
- Inhale. Exhaling, pull the heel back to the Base Position without moving your pelvis.
- Repeat with the other leg.

Variation:

- Inhale. Exhaling, slide your heel out; inhaling, pull your heel in. This variation is more demanding of core control.

  Caution: Avoid excessive tension. Focus your energy on targeted muscles. Do not clench the jaw or throat or elevate the shoulders. Soften the chest. If you feel a lot of tension in the upper thighs, stop and stretch out.

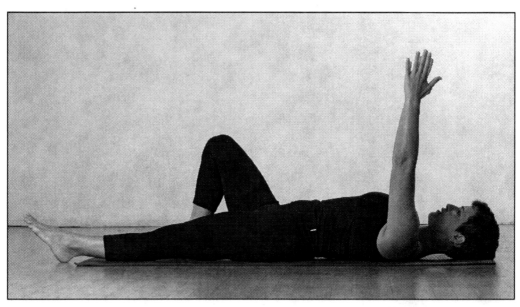

Figure 4.8
Leg slides

Note: Arms are elevated here to better show neutral spine. Arms are to be extended palms-down at your sides.

9. Curl-up with Long Arms (Articulating Curl-up)

• Lie supine in the Base Position with your arms extended palms-down at your sides.

• Exhaling, depress the scapulae to stabilize the shoulder girdle and open the chest. Gently draw the chin toward the chest as if holding an orange between the chin and the throat. Contract the abdominals and flex your upper body, with your fingertips reaching toward your ankles. Keep the pelvis in neutral position (Figure 4.9).

• Inhaling, roll down. Return the neck to neutral position.

Caution: If you have any neck pain or discomfort, try supporting the head with one hand, with the elbow out wide and the upper arm as flat as possible to keep the chest open. Switch the supporting hand, if necessary, for comfort. If you feel that you need to release any tension from the lower back, perform a Knee Hug Stretch (see page 37).

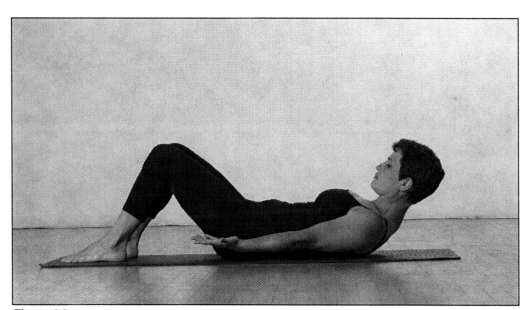

Figure 4.9
Curl-up with Long Arms

10. Chest Raise (Prone Cervical and Thoracic Extension)

- Lie prone with arms out, palms down, and elbows at 90 degrees. Together with the head, the arms form an "E" position. Rotate your thighs internally and contract your abdominal muscles to support a neutral pelvis (Figure 4.10a).
- Exhaling, elevate your upper body and arms without moving the pelvis, lengthening the spine upward (Figure 4.10b).

- Inhaling, lower to the starting position.

Variation:

To reduce intensity, keep your arms on the mat. Do not push the hands down as you lift; instead, simply rest your arms on the mat (Figure 4.11).

Caution: If you have back pain or discomfort or are unable to stabilize your pelvis, do not do this exercise. To stretch the abdominal and back muscles after this exercise, do the Shell Stretch and Cat Stretch (see pages 38 & 39).

Figure 4.10
Chest Raise

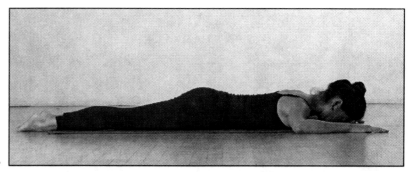

a.

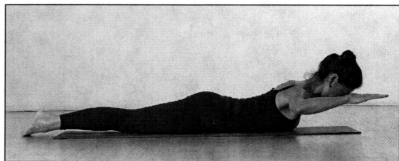

b.

Figure 4.10
Chest Raise—
variation

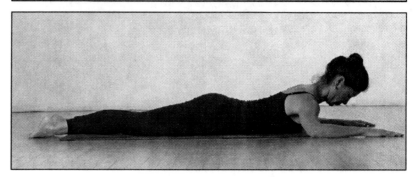

11. Leg Lifts (Prone Hip Extension)

• Lie prone, resting your head on your hands. Legs are long, with kneecaps touching the mat. Gently point your toes. Exhale; contract your abdominal muscles to establish neutral pelvis. Inhale as you prepare to move (Figure 4.12a).

• Exhale, keeping your pelvis stable and squeezing your buttocks, as you lift one leg off the mat. Be careful not to arch the back or flex the knees (Figure 4.12b).

• Inhaling, lower leg.

• Alternate legs with each repetition, or alternate sets using each leg.

Variation:

• When your abdominal and pelvic floor muscles are strong enough to stabilize the pelvis, lift both legs off the mat (Figure 4.13). Do not progress to this level until you are able to lift one leg 10 times without arching your back.

   Caution: Do not do this exercise if you feel lower-back pain or discomfort.

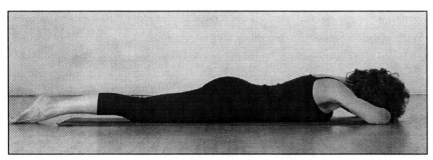

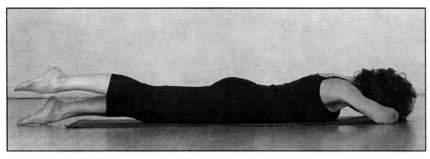

Figure 4.12
Leg Lifts

a.

b.

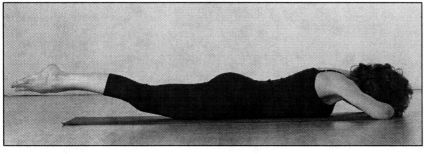

Figure 4.13
Leg Lifts—
variation

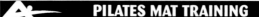

12. Knee Sways Stretch

    (Supine Spinal Rotation)

• Lie supine in the Base Position with your
  arms slightly angled out from your sides in
  an "A" position with palms up (Figure
  4.14a).

• Pull your knees and feet together.

• Inhale as you prepare to move.

• Exhale as you allow both legs to sway to one
  side, keeping your scapulae on the mat and
  knees flexed. Feel the stretch along the side

of your torso and in your lower back (Figure
4.14b).

• Inhale. Exhale as you pull your legs back to
  the center start position.

• Repeat, swaying your legs to the other side.

• Repeat, alternating sides.

Variation:

• After completing at least three repetitions side
  to side, you may hold your knees to one side for
  a static stretch for one to two breath cycles.

• Repeat on the other side.

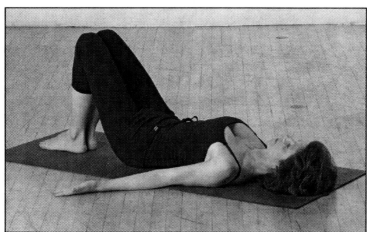

Figure 4.14
Knee Sways Stretch

a.

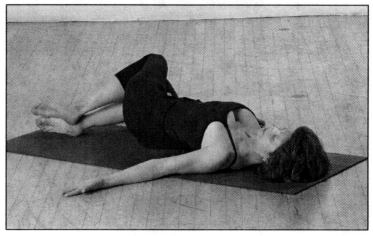

b.

13. Knee Hug Stretch

• Lie supine in the Base Position with your arms extended palms-down at your sides.

• Bring both knees toward your chest. Place your arms around the backs of your thighs. Avoid any pressure in the knees. Inhale as you hold the position (Figure 4.15).

• Exhale as you gently pull your knees toward your chest. Feel the stretch in your buttocks and lower back. Hold for 15 to 30 seconds.

Variation:

• For an inner-thigh stretch, pull your knees toward your shoulders. Feel the stretch in your inner thighs, buttocks, and lower back. Hold for 15 to 30 seconds (Figure 4.16).

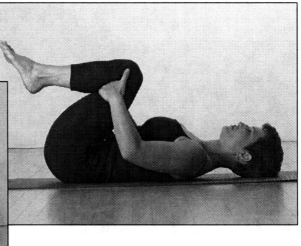

Figure 4.15
Knee Hug Stretch

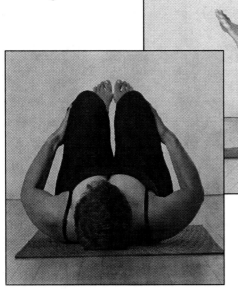

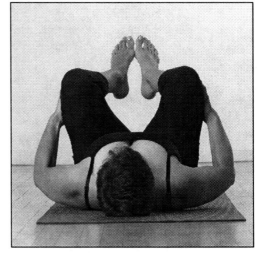

Figure 4.16
Knee Hug
Stretch—variation

14. Shell Stretch

• Start in an all-fours position.

• Exhale and lift your abdominal muscles as you create a posterior pelvic tilt and lower your hips toward your heels as far as is comfortable for your knees. Reach your arms forward, palms-down on the mat. Continue to breathe, and focus on expanding your rib cage with each inhalation and rounding your lower back with each exhalation (Figure 4.17). Hold for 15 to 30 seconds.

• To finish, lift your hips back up to the starting position.

   Caution: If you have any knee pain or discomfort, do not lower your hips completely to your heels. If this modification does not help, substitute the Knee Hug Stretch (see page 37).

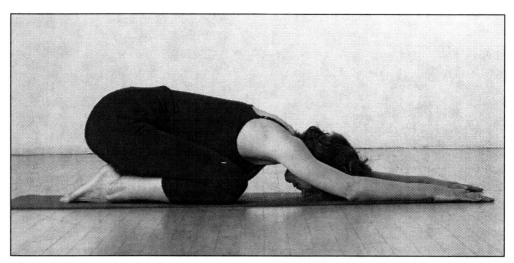

Figure 4.17
Shell Stretch

15. Cat Stretch (Quadruped Spine Flexion)

• Start in an all-fours position. Maintain neutral spinal alignment and lengthen through the neck and torso.

• Exhale as you flex your spine (Figure 4.18).

• Inhale as you return to the starting position.

• If your knees are uncomfortable in an all-fours position, substitute the Knee Hug Stretch (see page 37).

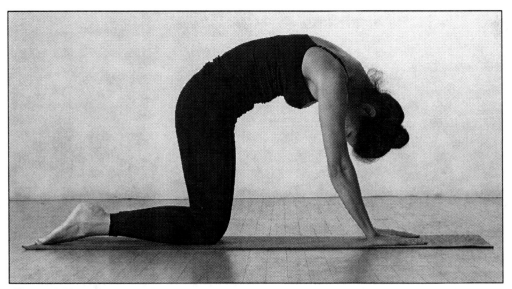

Figure 4.18
Cat Stretch

Core Stabilization

16. Modified Plank—Beginner

• Lie prone with your legs straight. Rest your forearms on the mat with your palms facing each other and your elbows directly beneath your shoulders. Depress your scapulae to stabilize the shoulders. Maintain neutral neck alignment (Figure 4.19).

• Contract your abdominal muscles to stabilize the torso and lift the rib cage. Do not arch your back. Work up to a 30-second hold.

Variations:

• To increase difficulty, lift thighs off the floor, maintaining length in your spine. Be sure your body weight is distributed between the elbows and forearms and the knees. Work up to a 30-second hold (Figure 4.20).

• To further increase difficulty, curl your toes under and push up onto your toes and the balls of your feet. Distribute your body weight between the elbows and forearms and the balls of your feet. Work up to a 30-second hold (Figure 4.21).

Caution: If you have any shoulder pain or discomfort, perform only the easiest version. To stretch the abdominal and back muscles after this exercise, do the Shell Stretch and Cat Stretch (see pages 38 & 39).

Figure 4.19
Modified Plank

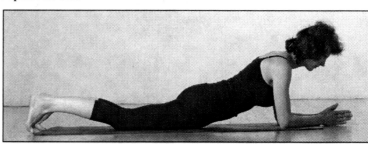

Figure 4.20
Modified Plank—
variation

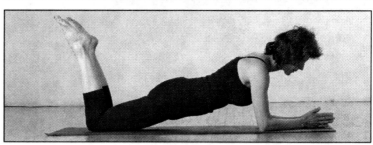

Figure 4.21
Modified Plank—
variation

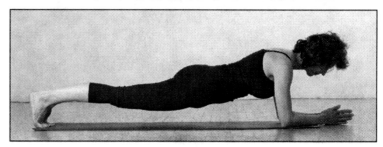

17. Modified Scapular Push-up (Quadruped Scapular Push-up)—Beginner

- Begin in an all-fours position with hands shoulder-width apart (Figure 4.22a).
- Inhaling, bend your elbows slightly and retract the scapulae (Figure 4.22b). (While the goal of achieving neutral posture requires a neutral thoracic position, retracting the scapulae enhances body awareness for the ultimate purpose of achieving scapular stability in neutral.)
- Exhaling, push up through the hands and protract the scapulae (Figure 4.22c).

Caution: If you have wrist pain or discomfort, place a rolled towel under your palms, allowing the fingers to touch the mat. Elevating your palms relieves wrist pressure. Place a towel under your knees for additional cushioning.

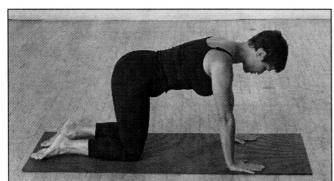

a.

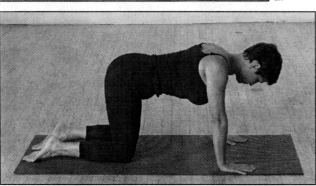

b.

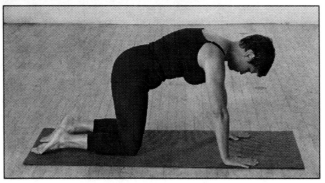

c.

Figure 4.22
Modified Scapular Push-up

18. Upward Facing Leg Pull, Prep (Modified Supine Plank)—Beginner

• Sit with your hands palms-down behind and outside of your hips, with your fingers facing whatever direction is most comfortable. Bend your knees and place your feet on the mat (Figure 4.23a).

• Exhale and push your feet into the mat as you lift the trunk upward into a "table" position. Contract your buttocks and hamstrings to lift the hips. Your hands should remain directly under the shoulders. Straighten your arms but avoid locking the elbows. Stabilize your shoulders and look straight ahead (Figure 4.23b).

Cautions: If you feel any wrist pain or discomfort, roll up a towel and place it under your palms, allowing your fingers to touch the mat. Elevating your palms relieves wrist pressure. To build strength for this exercise, practice the Modified Plank (see page 40).

If you experience discomfort in the neck, slowly move the head back to a more comfortable position.

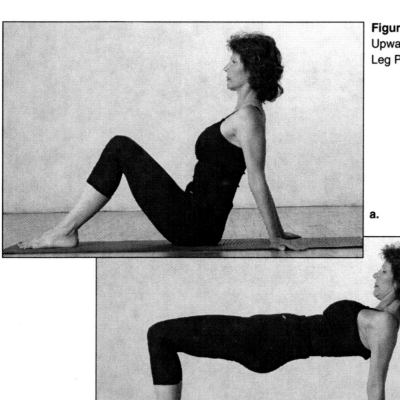

Figure 4.23
Upward Facing
Leg Pull, Prep

a.

b.

19. Side Bend Prep (Side Plank)—Beginner

• Begin in a side-lying position, with your bottom elbow under your shoulder, forearm and palm down, bottom knee flexed 90 degrees, top leg straight, and the top arm in front of the body (Figure 4.24a).

• Exhaling, lift your hip up off the mat, keeping the shoulder stabilized and sweeping the top arm straight up. Do not elevate your shoulder; keep your back and neck long. Contract your abdominal muscles and keep your buttocks contracted to stabilize the pelvis. Keep your chest and back wide (Figure 4.24b).

• Inhaling, lower your body back to the starting position. Keep your torso perpendicular to the mat. Do not rock forward or back.

• Repeat on the other side.

Caution: If you have shoulder pain or discomfort, do not do this exercise. Continue practicing the Modified Plank and Modified Scapular Push-up to build strength (see pages 40 & 41).

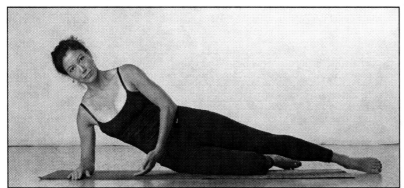

Figure 4.24
Side Bend Prep

a.

b.

20. Side Bend—Intermediate

• Begin in a side-lying position, with your chest open wide, pelvis perpendicular to the mat, bottom palm down on the mat under your shoulder, legs straight, and top arm in front of your body, palm up (Figure 4.25a).

• Exhaling, push into the mat with the hand and lift your hips and upper legs up into a neutral spine position as you sweep the top arm in an arc up and over your head. Stabilize your shoulders; keep your back and neck long; contract your abdominal muscles and keep your buttocks contracted to stabilize the pelvis. Do not collapse into the shoulder. Keep your chest and back wide (Figure 4.25b).

• Inhaling, lower your body back to the starting position. Keep your torso perpendicular to the mat and do not rotate your body forward or back.

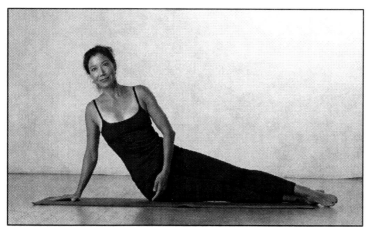

Figure 4.25
Side Bend

a.

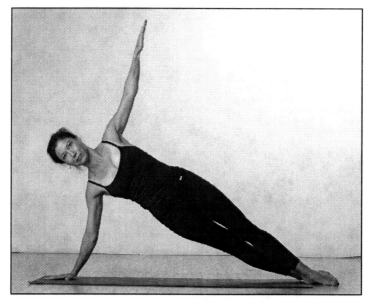

b.

21. Side Kick—Advanced

• Lie on your side and establish a neutral spine, with your pelvis perpendicular to the mat and your waist lifted. Rest your head on your outstretched arm, keeping your neck long. Place the top arm on the side of your ribs, flex your elbow 90 degrees, and place your hand on the mat in front of your navel like a kickstand. With your spine in neutral, lift the top leg to parallel to the floor (Figure 4.26a).

• Inhaling, dorsiflex the ankle of the top leg and bring it forward as far as possible, keeping the torso still (Figure 4.26b). Horizontally pulse the leg twice at the end of the range of motion. Do not rotate your torso forward or backward or lose neutral spine position.

• Exhaling, plantarflex the ankle of the top leg and pull the leg backward as far as possible without moving your torso. Keep your pelvis in neutral position (Figure 4.26c). Again, horizontally pulse the leg twice at the end of the range of motion.

• To finish, return the top leg to a position directly above the lower leg.

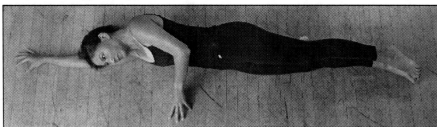

Figure 4.26
Side Kick

a.

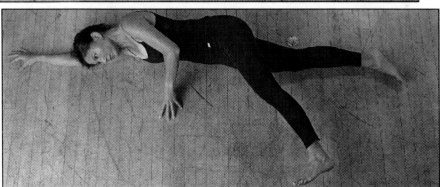

b.

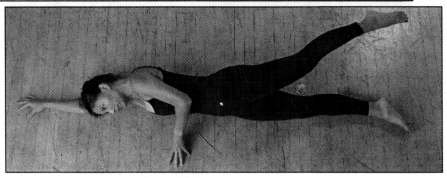

c.

Flexion

22. The Hundred I—Beginner

• Lie supine in the Base Position with your arms extended palms-down at your sides (Figure 4.27a).

• Inhaling, depress the scapulae to stabilize your shoulders and open your chest.

• Mildly contract your abdominal muscles. Exhaling, sequentially flex the cervical and thoracic spine up to curl off the mat, with your fingertips reaching toward your ankles. Hold the position.

• Pump your arms up and down five times while inhaling. Then, pump your arms up and down five times while exhaling (Figure 4.27b). Each breath cycle features 10 arm pumps, or beats.

• Repeat for 10 breath cycles, if possible. The 10 arm beats for 10 breath cycles equals 100 arm pumps, which is where this exercise gets its name.

Variation:

• As a reminder to keep the chest and back open, keep your palms up when inhaling and down when exhaling.

 Caution: If you have any neck pain or discomfort, support the head with one hand, with the elbow out wide and the upper arm as flat as possible to keep the chest open. Perform beats with the other arm. Switch hands after five breath cycles.

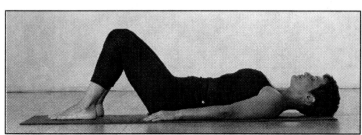

Figure 4.27
The Hundred I

a.

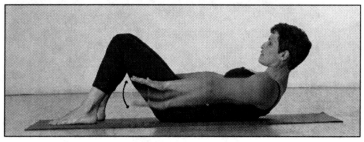

b.

23. The Hundred II—Intermediate to Advanced

- Lie supine in the Base Position with your arms extended palms-down at your sides. Lift your knees up above your hips. Extend one leg, then the other. Inhale; depress the scapulae to stabilize your shoulders and open your chest.

- Begin with legs held high in a vertical position. Maintain a neutral pelvis and lower the legs as strength permits. Avoid hyperextending the spine. If neutral pelvis cannot be maintained with the legs fully extended, bend the knees 90 degrees.

- Contract your abdominal muscles. Exhaling, curl up the upper spine, reaching your arms forward at shoulder height.

- Pump your arms up and down five times while inhaling (Figure 4.28). Then, pump your arms up and down five times while exhaling. Each breath cycle features 10 arm pumps, or beats.

- Repeat for 10 breath cycles.

Variation:

- As a reminder to keep an open chest and back, keep your palms up while inhaling and down while exhaling.

   Caution: If you have any neck pain or discomfort, try supporting the head with one hand, with the elbow out wide and the upper arm as flat as possible to keep the chest open. Perform beats with the other arm. Switch hands after five breath cycles.

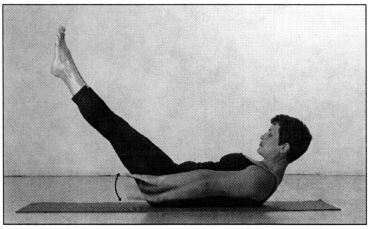

Figure 4.28
The Hundred II

24. Rolling Back—Beginner

• Sit on your ischium. Pull both knees toward your chest and gently point and place your toes on the mat for balance, and place one hand midway down each shin (Figure 4.29a).

• Exhaling, depress the scapulae, contract your abdominals, round the spine, and tilt your pelvis posteriorly so you are sitting just behind the ischium.

• Inhaling, roll back onto your shoulders, lifting the ischium toward the ceiling (Figures 4.29b & c).

• Exhaling, roll back up to the starting position, using your deep abdominal muscles to stop you before your toes touch the mat.

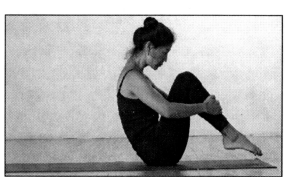

a.

Figure 4.29
Rolling Back

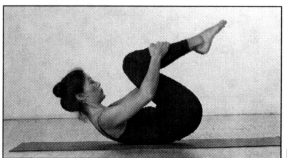

b.

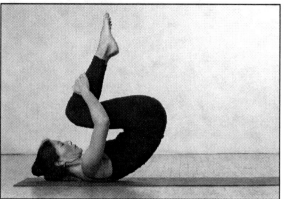

c.

Variation:

• If you are having trouble controlling your momentum, place your hands palms-down on either side of your hips. Use your hands to assist you as you roll back and up (Figure 4.30).

Cautions: Do not perform this exercise if you have osteoporosis. Do not roll on your neck or head. Do not do this exercise if you cannot control your momentum. If the lower back is contracted or rigid, you may be unable to tuck your pelvis under sufficiently to roll. If so, skip this exercise until you become more flexible. Instead, try the Knee Hug Stretch, Shell Stretch, and Cat Stretch (see pages 37, 38, & 39).

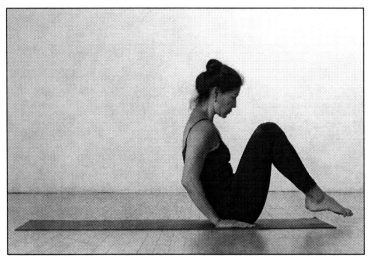

Figure 4.30
Rolling Back—variation

25. Single-leg Stretch—Beginner to Intermediate

- Lie supine in the Base Position with your arms extended palms-down at your sides.
- Exhaling, lift your right knee toward the chest with the shin parallel to the mat (Figure 4.31a).
- Exhaling, contract the deep abdominals. Feel your pelvis tilt posteriorly and the hip bones and rib cage move toward each other, shortening the waist and "imprinting" your spine on the mat.
- Inhale. Exhaling, curl the upper spine off the mat, reaching your right hand to the outside of your ankle and your left hand to the inside of your knee as you lift your right leg up to a 45-degree angle. Reestablish neutral pelvis if possible. Keep your elbows lifted and wide.

Figure 4.31
Single-leg Stretch

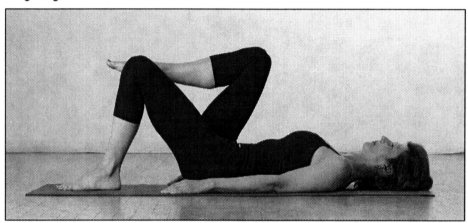

a.

• Inhale. Exhaling, switch legs, pulling one knee toward your chest while extending the other leg and switching hand positions. Keep your upper body lifted and the pelvis stabilized. Keep your abdominals contracted. Inhale as first one knee then the other comes toward your chest. Then, exhale as one knee then the other comes toward your chest (Figure 4.31b).

Caution: If you have neck or shoulder pain or discomfort, keep your upper body on the mat.

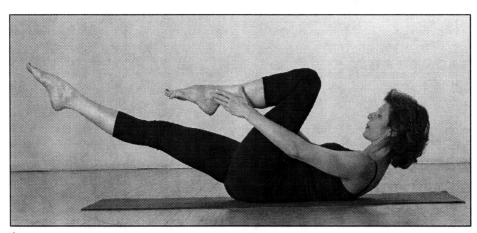

b.

26. Spine Stretch (Seated Spine Flexion)—
Beginner

• Sit with neutral spinal alignment and your legs straight, feet slightly wider than hip-width apart. Rest your hands between your legs, flex your feet, contract your abdominal muscles, and relax the shoulders (Figure 4.32a). If your pelvis tilts posteriorly, put a towel wedge under it to tilt it forward into neutral.

• Exhaling, leading with the top of the head, round the spine toward the pubic bone. Keep your abdominal muscles contracted to keep

Figure 4.32
Spine Stretch

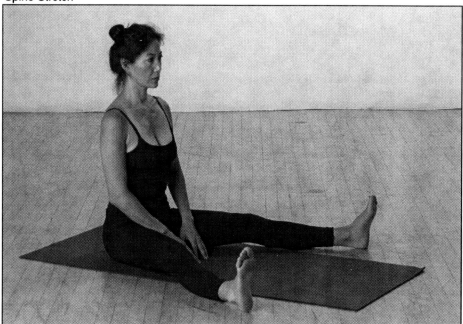

a.

the ischium in contact with the mat and to keep the pelvis in a vertical, neutral position. Slide your hands forward as flexibility permits (Figure 4.32b).

• Inhaling, hold this position, relaxing your back muscles into a stretch and keeping your abdominal muscles contracted. Breathe deeply.

• Exhaling, round your back up, stacking the vertebrae one at a time from the bottom up. Finish in a tall, neutral posture.

Variation:

• If the backs of your legs are tight, flex your knees slightly. Elevate the pelvis several inches above the mat by sitting on a pad or towel.

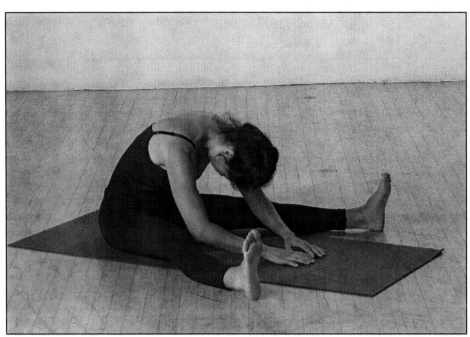

b.

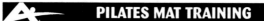
Extension

27. Swimming—Beginner to Advanced

• Lie prone with your legs straight and your kneecaps on the mat. Gently point your toes, lengthen the body, and stretch your arms out past your ears without elevating the shoulders (Figure 4.33a).

• Exhaling, contract your deep abdominal muscles to establish a neutral lower back.

• Inhale. Exhaling, simultaneously raise your arms parallel to the mat and lift your legs to approximately the same height. Your limbs should hover over the mat as high as possible while maintaining a neutral pelvis. Lengthen the body through the back of the neck (Figure 4.33b).

• Alternate lifting one arm and the opposite leg as if you are "swimming" (Figure 4.33c). Coordinate your breathing with the movement

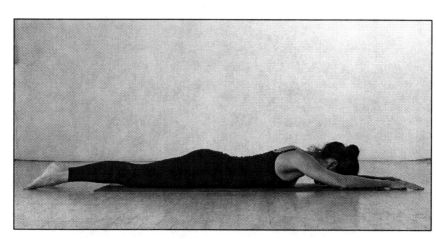

a.

Figure 4.33
Swimming

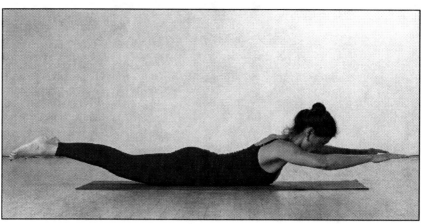

b.

by inhaling for five beats and exhaling for five beats, similar to The Hundred I breathing pattern (see page 46).

• Continue for five breath cycles, then lower your arms and legs back to the mat.

Variations:

• For an easier version, alternate lifting and lowering opposite arms and legs without hovering over the mat.

• To target the outer hips, rotate your legs so your heels fall internally and kneecaps face externally.

Caution: Avoid hyperextension of the lower back or neck. Stop if you have lower-back or shoulder pain or discomfort. To stretch the abdominal and back muscles after this exercise, do the Shell Stretch and Cat Stretch (see pages 38 & 39).

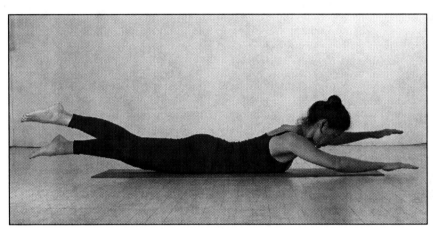

c.

28. Modified Swan Dive—Intermediate to Advanced

• Lie prone with your legs straight and feet shoulder-width apart. Externally rotate your legs, gently point your toes, and place your hands outside the shoulders, palms down (Figure 4.34a).

• Inhaling, stabilize your shoulders and use your back muscles to arc upward off the mat. Contract your abdominal muscles to avoid hyperextension of the lower back, and pull the rib cage internally. Keeping the back of the neck long, lift your upper body as high as possible while keeping your shoulders stable without elevating them (Figure 4.34b).

• Exhaling, rock your upper body forward and down, keeping your buttocks muscles contracted and lifting both legs as high as possible (Figure 4.34c).

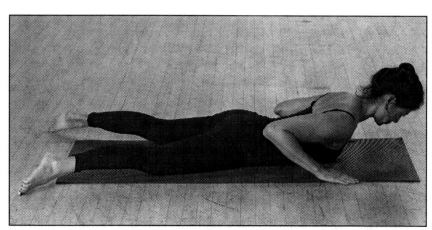

Figure 4.34
Modified
Swan Dive

a.

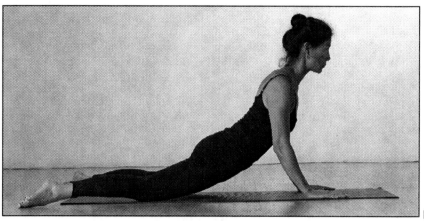

b.

• Continue alternating between the upper- and lower-body lift, five to eight times each.

Variation:

• When you have enough core strength to hold your body in an arc position: exhale and reach your arms forward in a "dive" (Figure 4.35). Keep them forward and inhale while rocking back onto your hips. To finish, place your hands on the mat in the starting position and lie prone.

Caution: Stop this exercise if you have shoulder or back pain or discomfort. Practice Chest Raise and Leg Lifts to build strength (see pages 34 & 35). Do the Shell Stretch and Cat Stretch to stretch afterward (see pages 38 & 39).

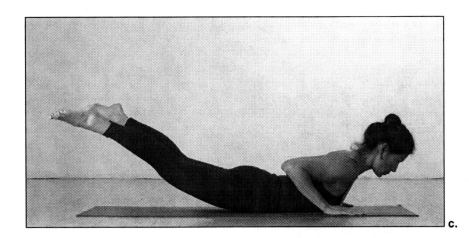

c.

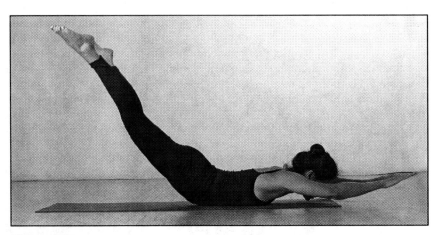

Figure 4.35
Modified Swan Dive—variation

Rotation

29. Spine Twist (Seated Spine Rotation)—
Beginner to Intermediate

• Sit with neutral spinal alignment and legs straight. Dorsiflex your feet, contract your abdominal muscles, stabilize your shoulders, and place your hands next to your hips (Figure 4.36a). If the pelvis tilts posteriorly, put a towel wedge under it to tilt it forward into neutral.

• Exhaling, lengthen your arms out straight to the sides, keeping your shoulders depressed (Figure 4.36b). Inhaling, lengthen the spine, lifting from the top of your head.

• Exhaling, rotate at the waist for two to three beats, moving slightly farther with each beat. The feet do not move and the pelvis remains down and facing forward. Do not swing your arms; instead, anchor the arms in place (Figure 4.36c).

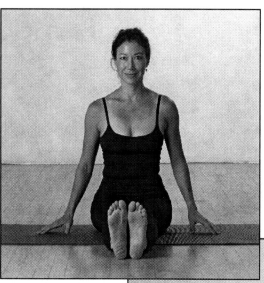

a.

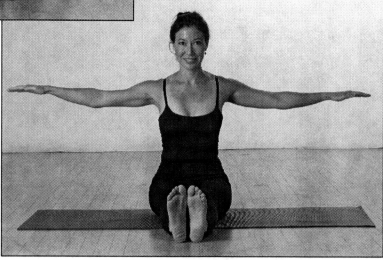

b.

Figure 4.36
Spine Twist

• Inhaling, return to center.

• Repeat in the opposite direction.

Variations:

• If the backs of your legs are tight, flex your knees slightly or sit in a cross-legged position.

• If it is not possible to keep your arms anchored when they are fully lengthened, shorten the lever length. Instead, touch the pads of your thumbs and fingers together, forming a tent-like shape with your hands. Touch the tips of your thumbs to your breastbone with your elbows out to the sides and shoulders depressed, then perform the remainder of the exercise as described above (Figure 4.37).

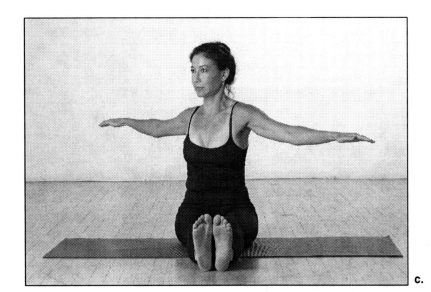

c.

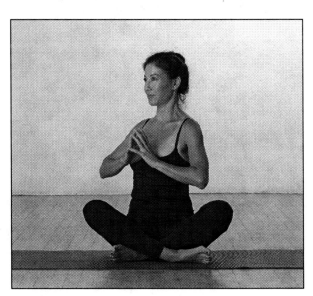

Figure 4.37
Spine Twist—variation

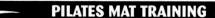
30. Crisscross (Supine Single-leg Stretch with Trunk Rotation)—Intermediate to Advanced

- Lie supine in the Base Position with your fingertips behind your head, elbows out wide, and shoulders depressed.
- Exhaling, lift one knee, then the other above your hip joints at 90 degrees. Inhale. Exhaling, rotate the upper body to the left, lifting your right shoulder toward the left knee. Draw the left knee in and extend the right leg at a 45-degree angle (Figure 4.38a).
- Inhale. Exhaling, switch legs and rotate each shoulder toward the opposite knee; maintain the lift in your upper body (Figure 4.38b). Contract the abdominal muscles to stabilize your pelvis. Avoid pulling on your neck.
- To finish, hug both knees to your chest and lower your upper body.

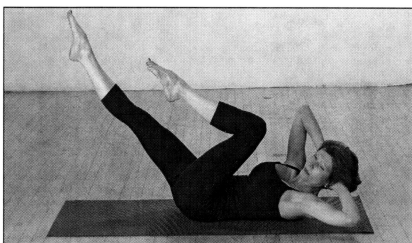

Figure 4.38
Crisscross

a.

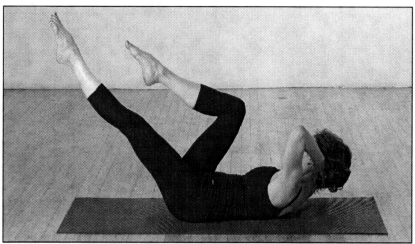

b.

Variation:

• If you are unable to stabilize the pelvis, place both feet on the mat with your knees flexed 90 degrees. Exhaling, rotate the shoulder toward the opposite knee (Figure 4.39).

Inhaling, roll down through center. Continue, alternating sides.

Caution: If you have neck or shoulder pain or discomfort, keep your upper body on the mat or skip this exercise altogether.

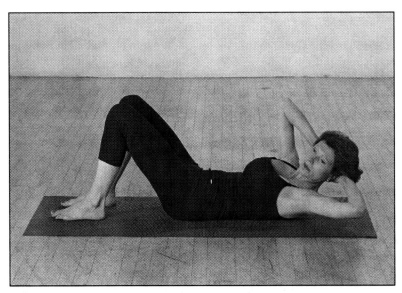

Figure 4.39
Crisscross—variation

Sequencing

When designing a workout sequence, it is important to: include a warm-up; consider the ease with which one exercise flows naturally into another according to body position; provide a variety of flexion, extension, and rotation exercises for balanced muscular development; and provide rest for certain muscle groups. For example, depending on the muscular endurance of your participants, you may have more than one flexion exercise in a row. However, if your participants do not have sufficient muscle endurance to perform a series of flexion exercises, then it is best to alternate them with extension and rotation exercises.

Sample Workout

The following sequence constitutes a balanced Pilates mat workout. Repeat each exercise five to 10 times, depending on the individual exercise. For final stretches, include those that release the muscles of the back, hip flexors, buttocks, abdomen, chest, shoulders, neck, inner and outer thighs, and the sides of the trunk.

1. Base Position
2. Pilates Breathing
3. Pelvic Clock
4. Pelvic Tilt
5. Bridge
6. Shoulder Slaps
7. Bridge (Rib Cage Arms Variation)
8. Knee Sways Stretch
9. Curl-up with Long Arms
10. The Hundred I or II
11. Modified Plank
12. Shell Stretch
13. Cat Stretch
14. Single-leg Stretch
15. Crisscross
16. Modified Scapular Push-up
17. Chest Raise
18. Shell Stretch
19. Leg Lifts
20. Modified Swan Dive
21. Rolling Back
22. Spine Stretch
23. Spine Twist
24. Side Bend Prep or Side Bend
25. Final Stretches

CHAPTER FIVE

Teaching Pilates Mat Exercises

Because the Pilates method works well for both personal training and group instruction, the teaching techniques discussed in this chapter are applicable to both, with the exception of the information that pertains to instructor-to-student ratios and class levels. Joseph Pilates himself taught in both one-on-one and group settings.

Pre-screening

Ideally, if you are teaching group classes, all of the participants will have been pre-screened by the facility that is offering the program according to fitness industry standards and guidelines. To provide safe instruction, you must be aware of any pre-existing health conditions. Personal trainers usually have more individual control over this process and should observe standard pre-screening practices.

If you learn of any musculoskeletal disorders through the pre-screening process that require the attention of a healthcare professional, refer the individual for a medical release. Even though Pilates is used for rehabilitation, it is essential that you stay within your scope of practice and only teach what you have learned through appropriate training and only to clients whom you are qualified to work with.

Instructor-to-Student Ratio and Class Levels

While the number of students that a group fitness instructor can handle varies according to his or her experience and skill level, most experts agree that Pilates mat classes should be smaller in size than the typical group exercise class. The recommended maximum number of students ranges from as few as six to as many as 16. The instructor-to-student ratio is significant because Pilates is meant to be a highly supervised form of movement.

As an instructor, you need to be able to observe closely the performance of each participant and to offer individual modifi-

cations as appropriate. Precision, control, and movement quality are hallmarks of the Pilates method; therefore, a good instructor is constantly guiding participants on movement form and alignment. Newer instructors may only be able to handle up to eight participants.

For this reason, many health and fitness facilities prefer to offer small Pilates mat classes on a fee basis. This not only regulates the class size through enrollment, but also permits continuous progressive training. Often participants understand that becoming a qualified Pilates instructor requires an investment of time and money in specialty training and are willing to pay for the instruction accordingly. In addition, most successful program directors agree that maintaining high-quality standards is essential to the long-term success of a Pilates program.

Students will progress on their learning curve over time so class levels are also important. While it is not as difficult to merge inter-mediate and advanced participants, it is challenging to provide a safe, effective, and efficient workout to a group that includes both beginners and advanced exercisers. New partic-ipants, regardless of how fit they are, need to learn the foundation moves and essential principles of Pilates, so they can comprehend how Pilates training is different from other forms of exercise. People with high levels of body awareness and conditioning will advance rapidly to more difficult levels, while others may spend more time mastering the basics. Some form of introductory training is essential so exercisers will understand the importance of working at their own individual level at al times and of not copying other participants in a group.

Workout Components

Pilates exercise is classified as a mind-body exercise and must be taught accordingly. Nonetheless, it is no different than any other type of physical training in terms of the need to ensure safety by providing an activity-specific warm-up, appropriate modifications and progressions for movements, and an activity-specific cool-down.

Warm-up

Similar to other exercise formats, the purpose of the Pilates mat workout warm-up is to prepare the exerciser both physically and mentally for the upcoming session. Exercisers perform most Pilates mat exercises from a lying position on the mat; however, you can warm up clients in either a standing or lying position. As with all workout sessions, the warm-up will vary depending on the time of day and the environment. For example, an early-morning session requires a more vigorous rhythmic warm-up to stimulate blood circulation and lubrication of the joints. In contrast, a late-day session's warm-up could include deep breathing, gentle stretching, and progressively more vigorous exercises. All warm-ups should be at least five to eight minutes long, depending on the condition of the participants.

Because Pilates is a form of mind-body movement, the warm-up should not only physically prepare the individual, but also mentally transition the client to an inner awareness of the mind-body connection. Include breathing exercises, or breath awareness, combined with attention to alignment, from the start of the training session. In addition, include exercises that mobilize the major joints of the body such as the spine, neck, shoulders, hips, and knees, to stimulate the flow of synovial fluid and to prepare the body for more rigorous exercises.

The warm-up is an ideal time to review each of the Pilates principles—concentration, control, physical centering, flowing movement, precision, and breathing—to mentally prepare clients for the Pilates approach, while physically going through the foundation exercises. For beginners, you can design the entire session around foundation movements. To train experienced participants, organize the workout using foundation exercises as a warm-up.

An integral aspect of Pilates practice is re-educating movement patterns of the body as a whole. Therefore, the warm-up is also an ideal opportunity to review concepts of synergistic movement. For example, begin with standing balance exercises to heighten awareness of proprioception, or with forms of total-body movements that do not place undue emphasis on isolated parts.

The warm-up also is the ideal time to review the Base Position, to ensure everyone understands the concept of neutral alignment, and to reinforce the importance of using good body mechanics throughout the workout. This is the time to check in with all the participants to see how they are doing and if they have any information about their physical condition to share. You determine how all of these elements are blended in an individual warm-up. The successful teaching of Pilates, as it is with many movement disciplines and sports, is as much art as science.

Exercises for Peak Training

The level of difficulty of the exercises is determined by the abilities of the participants. In a mixed-level group, it is ideal to offer a variety of options for each exercise and to create an atmosphere that encourages people to select individually appropriate exercises. Every workout, regardless of level, should include a variety of flexion, extension, and rotation movements for a balanced workout.

For example, a more advanced group can perform multiple flexion exercises in a row. Sequencing exercises in this manner provides a challenge in a way that is similar to the concept of a super set or giant set, where the same muscle group is stimulated in slightly different ways to elicit a training response.

Cool-down

The specific cool-down for a contemporary Pilates mat session should be structured to match the intensity level of the activities. For example, a more advanced group that moves at a faster pace with more vigor may require a longer cool-down segment than a low-intensity, introductory-level session. An ideal use of the cool-down time is to stretch particularly tight muscles that have been warmed up during the workout.

For example, many exercisers who have a kyphotic-lordotic posture will have tight lower-back muscles, hip flexors, internal obliques, shoulder adductors, and intercostals. Therefore, more time can be allocated during the cool-down to stretching these areas. The cool-down also provides an opportunity to focus on breathing. Ideally, the cool-down should last anywhere from three to 10 minutes, depending on the length of the training session and the needs of the participants.

Cueing

Successful cueing for Pilates mat exercises is critically important for the client to have a positive experience and to achieve the mind-body connection. Quality of form, alignment, movement flow, and breathing all need to be directed in as few words as possible. Characteristic qualities of mindful exercise include attention to the present moment, focusing on the process rather than performance goals, emphasis on breathing, and self-awareness. Good cueing can ensure that these mindful qualities are present in every session.

Voice quality is more important in a mind-body style of class than in other classes, as it can greatly impact the mood of a session. Use a relaxing but confident tone and avoid over-vocalization. While it is important to cue, it is also important not to overwhelm participants. Appropriate cueing can create a positive experience, motivate and inspire participants, and foster feelings of success and the desire to return again.

Use cueing to create a non-competitive atmosphere and help to ensure a safe exercise environment. With each exercise, it is a good idea to name the exercise and its purpose. Depending on the experience level of the group, it may be appropriate to demonstrate the exercise. Cues should guide the exerciser from the starting position and explain clearly how the breath coordinates with the movement. Provide modifications as necessary and encourage participants to choose whatever level is appro-priate for their abilities. Clearly explain any common errors or risks related to faulty execution, so exercisers can avoid injury.

The use of visualizations can be an effective method of cueing to assist clients in imagining a total-body feeling or experience. You need to be very comfortable with the choice of visual-izations so that the proper effect is created. Take time to develop personal visualizations and practice recording and listening back to your cues. Time invested in this manner will yield tremendous improvements.

Evaluate the necessity of hands-on cueing with care. Some clients do not want to be touched, and certain states do not allow trainers to physically touch clients. If touch is necessary, a prop can be used to administer the cue, as in touching someone while holding a ball in your hand to avoid direct contact. While some experts insist that physical touch is an essential part of teaching the Pilates method, you still need to exercise caution and good judgment. Some individuals may construe touching as a form of sexual harassment. Use discretion and always ask permission prior to touching any participants. A simple question—"May I touch your shoulder to help teach you the movement?"—will let you know how comfortable the individual is with touching.

Use of Props

The only item other than a mat that is essential for a Pilates mat exercise program is a towel, which provides additional cushioning and absorbs perspiration. If participants have muscular tightness in the neck, upper back, and shoulders, suggest that they put a rolled or folded towel under the head to maintain neutral neck alignment. In side-lying positions, clients use a towel as a pillow under the head or place it under the waist for additional support.

Other popular props for mat exercises include the "magic circle," or fitness circle, a small ball, a foam roller, and a stability ball (Figure 5.1). If any additional props are incorporated, it is essential to receive proper training on use. When props are introduced into workouts, sequencing should continue to be smooth with a minimal amount of disruption. Always observe each manufacturer's suggested instructions for storage and care.

Choosing a Mat

Pilates mat exercises differ from other forms of exercise in that they often involve rolling on the back or on the stomach. These rolling movements are much more comfortable with adequate cushioning, particularly for participants who do not have a lot of natural padding on their bodies. On the other hand, a mat that is too soft makes it difficult for exercisers to tell whether or not they are maintaining neutral spinal alignment when lying down. An exerciser requires some firmness under the

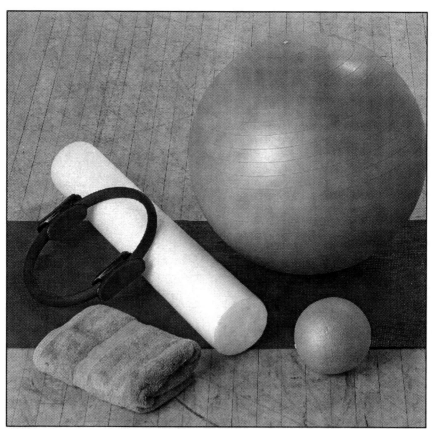

Figure 5.1
Props commonly used in Pilates mat training

spine to be able to distinguish the natural curves of the spine from points of contact on the mat.

The ideal mat is made of a rubber-like material and is at least ⅜-inch thick. A ⅛-inch thick yoga "sticky mat" is generally too thin for Pilates practice. The typical firm, dense foam mats used for group exercise may be too hard for comfort and too short to accommodate the entire body in a prone or supine position.

Mat Cleaning

Mat hygiene is important. If you are teaching in a facility that provides mats to participants, encourage exercisers to use a towel on top of the mat. Ideally, if clients make a commitment to practicing regularly, encourage them to purchase their own mat. For shared mats, check the manufacturer's instructions for appropriate cleaning procedures. Some high-priced mats are made with antibacterial materials to help offer protection against transferable infections.

Space and Environment Requirements

When performing Pilates mat exercises, exercisers need enough space to stand up, lie down, reach the arms overhead and around the body, and lift their legs up and to the sides of the body. In an ideal group exercise setting, each participant is positioned at least a leg-length apart. The floor surface should be firm (either wood or industrial carpet is appropriate) and the floor space should be clear and free from clutter. The exercise classroom should have mirrors on at least two of its four walls as recommended by the facility standards and guidelines of the American College of Sports Medicine (1997). Mirrors allow interested participants to observe their movements for self-correction and increase your ability to see all participants.

Appropriate temperature, humidity, and air circulation levels are similar to those provided for muscle conditioning, flexibility, yoga, or tai chi classes. Moderately warmer temperatures [68 to 72° F (20 to 22° C)] are appropriate for beginning or less strenuous sessions.

An appropriate level of light allows participants to easily view the instructor. Because participants perform many exercises in a supine position, some experts suggest full spectrum light, as it is more comfortable on the eyes. Alternatively, you can slightly dim the lights or advise participants to position themselves so that they are not directly beneath an overhead light.

An important aspect of Pilates mat exercise is concentration, so the ideal environment will not have a lot of disruptive outside noises. Because this is not always possible in a fitness facility environment, music can assist in masking these outside noises. Keep studio doors closed and, if possible, schedule classes so as not to compete with other loud activities.

Attire

Guidelines for Pilates attire relate more to comfort than to safety. When performing mat exercises, participants need to be able to move easily and without restriction. Pilates mat exercises are low-impact; therefore, athletic bras and shoes are not essential. In fact, performing exercises barefoot makes it easier for feet to connect with the floor and helps to prevent slipping. Participants should wear either loose- or form-fitting apparel according to personal preference. Form-fitting clothes do not interfere with movement and make it easier for you to observe alignment. Pants with soft, wide waistbands and unitards with no waistband are the most comfortable garments for performing exercises in the supine position. Avoid clothing with buttons, snaps, or zippers that could rub or chafe.

Music

Music provides a soothing environment and can enhance participants' focus. While musical preferences are always subjective, many expert practitioners recommend instrumental music played in the background. However, other Pilates trainers use a variety of classical, jazz, new age, and even pop music. Music without a strong rhythmic beat can help participants to work at their own pace.

Progressions and Modifications

Pilates mat exercises can be modified to increase or decrease intensity as appropriate. You can create modifications by altering one or more of the following variables: base of support, lever length, range of motion, speed, number of repetitions, and use of props. Another strategy to modify an exercise and reduce intensity is to break down a complex, coordinated movement into simpler steps. Once the client has mastered the individual parts, the exercise can be reintegrated into a single, flowing movement.

For example, the Hundred II (see page 47) is executed with both legs elevated and extended with the upper body held in a flexed position for 10 breath cycles. This movement can be adapted to suit a variety of levels from beginning to advanced (Figures 5.2–5.7, pages 72–73). Of course, modifications made for an individual need to be based on a variety of factors including postural issues, muscular imbalances, and any physical limitations.

You need to thoroughly understand appropriate intensity modifications so that exercises can be kept safe for participants. The proper modification is one that provides the exerciser with a sense of challenge while still being able to control the movement and stabilize the core.

Injury Prevention

Your two most important responsibilities are to ensure effectiveness and safety. You can minimize the risk of injury during Pilates mat exercises by paying close attention to the following points:

• effective pre-screening

• close observation of exercise execution

• thorough cueing of each exercise

• modifications to suit individual ability

• reminders to work at an appropriate level

• teaching clients body awareness and how to self-monitor

• appropriate exercise progression

• requiring trainer approval for individual participation in advanced mat classes

All exercises that challenge postural stabilizers must be executed with care to avoid injury, especially to the neck, shoulders, back, and hips. You can minimize the likelihood of injury by observing the historical Pilates principles—concentration, control, physical centering, flowing movement, precision, and breathing—and by ensuring that any movements taught to clients are biomechanically sound and appropriate for each individual's level of fitness and Pilates expertise.

Figure 5.2
Keep the head
and both feet on
the mat

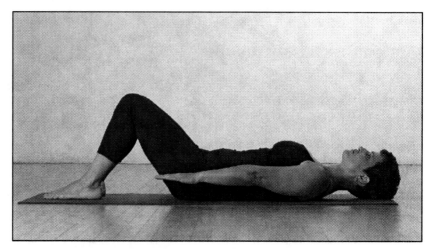

Figure 5.3
Elevate the head
and keep both feet
on the mat

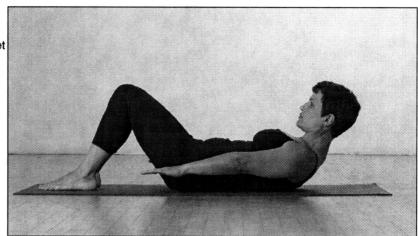

Figure 5.4
Elevate the
head, lift one leg
with the knee
flexed, and keep
one foot on the
mat

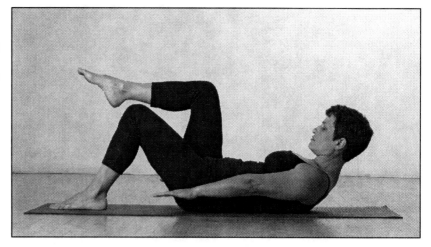

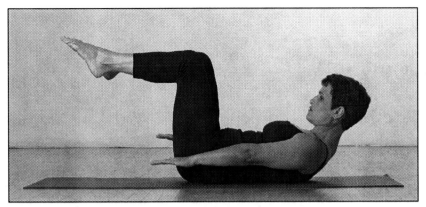

Figure 5.5
Elevate the head and lift both legs with the knees flexed

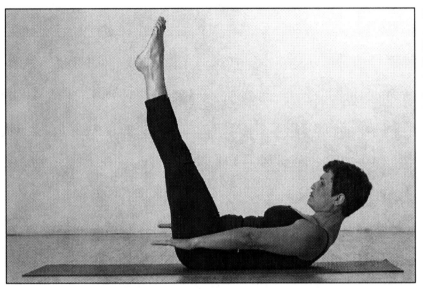

Figure 5.6
Elevate the head and lift both legs with the knees extended and legs held high

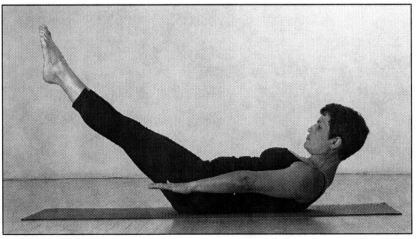

Figure 5.7
Elevate the head and lift both legs with the knees extended at approximately 45 degrees

Special

Populations

Pilates mat exercises are suitable for many people — male and female, old and young, deconditioned and elite athlete. The key to successful program design is to have the appropriate training to adapt exercises to the special needs of individual clients. Before working with any member of a special population group, you should be thoroughly trained regarding physical activity guidelines for that individual's needs.

Children

Children in America today need to increase daily physical activity, as the incidence of obesity and juvenile diabetes continue to rise. Mind-body exercise programs have been finding success with children as young as five or six years of age. Due to the need for concentration required of many of the exercises, however, the most successful programs have been with children age 11 and older. As with any children's movement activity, exercise sessions need to be shorter in length and fun in nature.

Physical modifications of exercises for children primarily center around preventing any undue stress or pressure on the spine, especially the cervical spine. Young people are still growing and their bones are not fully formed. Select exercises with care to avoid any stress on the spine, and particularly avoid flexion with any weightbearing on the upper back or in a side-lying position with the head resting on the hand.

Other safety precautions for children are the same as for adults. Cue children to breathe properly, to move with control, to avoid competition, and to avoid movements that cause undue discomfort or pain. Encourage children to drink plenty of fluids, and always give positive, supportive, corrective feedback.

Pre- and Post-natal

The guidelines set forth by the American College of Obstetricians and Gynecologists (ACOG) for safe and effective exercise during pregnancy apply to pregnant women who practice Pilates mat exercises (2002; 1994). Keep in mind that pregnancy is not a time to increase exercise, but rather a time to simply follow a maintenance program. All pre- and post-natal women should consult with their healthcare provider before participating in any exercise program. You may not be aware of continuing students who may become pregnant while training under your supervision; therefore, it is a good idea to announce that you also need to know if anyone is pregnant when asking about injuries.

The regular practice of Pilates mat exercises provides the following benefits to pre- and post-natal women:
• conditions abdominal, back, and pelvic floor muscles for greater support and stabilization
• enhances body awareness
• improves sense of balance, which is challenged as body size and shape change
• increases the mind-body connection and improves breath control, both of which can help the mother during labor

To reap the benefits of Pilates during pregnancy, however, it is important to observe certain precautions. In general, no exercises should be performed in the supine position after the first trimester. Instead, choose seated, all-fours, or side-lying positions. Exercises normally done in a prone position can be modified to an all-fours position. Pregnant women must avoid staying in any one position for a prolonged period of time due to circulatory challenges from increased body fluids and the needs of the growing fetus, so the ideal workout design includes frequent positional changes.

Remind pregnant clients to breathe. Holding the breath in or out can increase intra-abdominal pressure and reduce the oxygen supply to the fetus. Exercises such as the Shell Stretch and Cat Stretch are valuable to relieve tension in the lower back (see pages 38 & 39). Remind pregnant and postpartum clients who are still breastfeeding that the hormone relaxin continues to circulate in their bloodstream. Therefore, stretches need to be performed conservatively, only to a point of moderate tension with the stretch felt in the muscles and not in the joints.

Encourage pre- and post-natal exercisers to perform Kegels throughout their workouts to continue to strengthen the pelvic floor muscles. As with all Pilates mat exercises, the participant should activate the pelvic floor when contracting the deep abdominal muscles. For pregnant women, this is even more important as the pelvic floor muscles are stressed by the weight of the growing fetus.

Avoid spinal rotation exercises such as the Crisscross (see page 60). These exercises stress the oblique muscles and may contribute to diastasis recti, or a separation of the rectus abdominis muscle from the linea alba. After the first trimester other spinal flexion exercises will not be possible due to the increasing size of the fetus and are not recommended due to the stress on the rectus abdominis. Instead, emphasize exercises that focus on core stabilization and activation of the deep abdominals and pelvic floor.

Spinal extension exercises also pose risks for pregnant exercisers. For more detailed information regarding pre- and post-natal exercise see the ACE Guide for Fitness Professionals, *Pre- and Post-Natal Fitness*, by Lenita Anthony.

Deconditioned and Larger-sized

Never make assumptions about the physical conditioning or abilities of your participants based on size alone. Adaptations for exercises should be recommended on an individual basis depending on specific needs. For people who are deconditioned and who have excess body fat, it is common for the following postural deviations to be present:

• lordosis of the lumbar spine
• kyphosis of the thoracic spine accompanied by compression of the ribcage into the abdominal area
• flat, pronated feet

• compression of the leg joints

A balanced program of stretching, stabilization, and strengthening exercises can begin to address muscular imbalances.

Take positive steps to foster a supportive environment to encourage all participants regardless of size or level of ability. For example:

• reinforce the fact that everyone is successful simply for showing up

• remind everyone that any participation is positive

• encourage all participants to work at their own pace

• respect privacy

• consider offering classes in rooms where mirrors are optional, or remind clients that it is not necessary to look in the mirror if it is not comfortable

• when teaching a group class, be sure to face the class, and start each exercise at the lowest level and offer progressively more difficult options

• emphasize the discovery of the simple joy of movement

• find the fun in the activity

• use positive language to encourage clients to reconnect with their bodies

• use non-judgmental language to reinforce the fact that everyone can perform the exercises to the best of his or her own ability and still receive benefits

Keep in mind that additional body weight can reduce range of motion and, depending on where the weight is distributed, affect movement dynamics. For example, if someone has a larger upper body and a relatively smaller lower body, spinal flexion exercises from a supine position are relatively more difficult than for a person who has a small upper body and a heavier lower body. To maintain a positive environment, be ready to offer modifications. These can include performing an exercise with a reduced range of motion, starting from a seated position instead of a supine position, or performing exercises such as push-ups and certain stretches in a standing position using the wall for support.

When teaching floorwork, provide cues on how to get down to, and up from, the floor. Some larger-sized people may be too intimidated to lie on the floor because they lack confidence in their ability to get up. Knowing how to cue these movements can remove this concern. Use the following cues.

To get down to the floor:

Begin with a wide stance and put your hands on your thighs. Squat, and while bending your knees, lower one knee to the floor, extend a hand out, and lower your hips to the side on the floor.

To get up from the floor:

With your hands on the floor, assume a wide stance with both knees and your toes on the floor and heels up. Walk hands in, push off with hands, and roll weight into the heels. Continue to walk your hands up to your thighs, and push up to a standing position.

For participants who experience knee pain, provide alternatives for exercises in the quadruped position such as lying in a completely prone position or, in the case of the Shell Stretch or Cat Stretch (see pages 38 & 39), performing the Knee Hug Stretch as a knee-friendly alternative (see page 37). Final stretches can also be performed in a seated position on chairs.

Older Adults

The non-impact, lower-intensity nature of Pilates may be particularly attractive to older adults. In addition to these features, Pilates provides significant mental and physical benefits to older adult practitioners because of the cognitive focus and the emphasis on breath and body awareness. Pilates also offers valuable training to improve posture, coordination, and balance. Older adults, however, have a higher risk of injury, particularly when it comes to spinal movement and joint issues. Therefore, specialized training to understand how to suggest appropriate modifications is essential.

Some of the more common conditions that affect older adult participants include hypertension, heart disease, and arthritis. Exercises should be performed at a lower intensity and, when working with deconditioned participants, for shorter duration. Many older adults are on multiple medications that can affect their response to exercise. For example, deep breathing may adversely affect those on hypertension medications and lead to feelings of lightheadedness or dizziness. Thorough screening and a health history and medical release, if indicated, are therefore essential.

Osteoporosis

The prevalence of osteoporosis in the American population is increasing as the population continues to age. According to the National Osteoporosis Foundation, in 2002 55% of people age 50 and older had reduced bone density or osteoporosis. Of that group, more than 20% had osteoporosis, 80% of whom were women. Between the ages of 50 and 59 years of age, 37% of women had osteoporosis; and 87% of women age 80 years and older had osteoporosis. One of the more serious consequences of osteoporosis is the severity of bone fractures in the event of a fall. If the current rates of osteoporosis continue, one-half of women and one-fourth of men age 50 years and older will have an osteoporosis-related fracture in their lifetime. As many as 24% of hip-fracture patients age 50 and older die in the year following the fracture (National Osteoporosis Foundation, 2004).

The consequences of osteoporosis can be very serious; therefore, it is important that anyone with this condition have a medical release before engaging in any physical activity. While weightbearing exercises can slow the onset or deter the progression of this disease, they also present certain risks. In particular, spinal flexion should be avoided, as well as any forceful rotational movements. Hyperextension is also not appropriate. Because all of the Pilates mat exercises, except for those focusing on core stabilization in a neutral position, involve these movements, specific clearance is recommended.

American College of Obstetricians and Gynecologists (2002). *ACOG Committee Opinion: Exercise during Pregnancy and the Postpartum Period*. Washington, D.C.: American College of Obstetricians and Gynecologists.

American College of Obstetricians and Gynecologists (1994). *ACOG Technical Bulletin, #189*. Washington, D.C.: American College of Obstetricians and Gynecologists.

American College of Sports Medicine (1997). *ACSM's Health/Fitness Facility Standards and Guidelines* (2nd ed.). Champaign, Ill.: Human Kinetics.

American Council on Exercise (2003). *ACE Personal Trainer Manual* (3rd ed.). San Diego, Calif.: American Council on Exercise.

American Council on Exercise (2000). *Group Fitness Instructor Manual*. San Diego, Calif.: American Council on Exercise.

American Council on Exercise (1998). *Exercise for Older Adults*. Champaign, Ill.: Human Kinetics.

Anderson, B.D. & Spector, A. (2000). Introduction to Pilates-based rehabilitation. *Orthopaedic Physical Therapy Clinics of North America, 9*, 395–410.

Anthony, L. (2002). *Pre- and Post-Natal Fitness*. San Diego, Calif.: American Council on Exercise.

Archer, S. (2004). *Pilates Fusion: Well-Being for Body, Mind, and Spirit*. San Francisco, Calif: Chronicle Books.

Archer, S. (2003). *The Pilates Deck.*

San Francisco, Calif.: Chronicle Books.

Archer, S. (2001). Pilates trademark. *IDEA Health & Fitness Source, 11.*

Barlow, C.E. et al. (1995). Physical fitness, mortality and obesity. *International Journal of Obesity, 19*, S4, S41–44.

Benson, H. (1985). *Beyond the Relaxation Response*. New York, N.Y.: Berkley Books.

Benson, H. (1975). *The Relaxation Response*. New York, N.Y.: Avon Books.

Blair, N. & Paffenbarger, R.S. (1994). *Influence of Body Weight and Shape Variation on Incidence of Cardiovascular Disease, Diabetes, Lung Disease and Cancer*. Harvard Alumni Data: Paper presented at the 34th Annual Conference on Cardiovascular Disease, Epidemiology and Prevention, March 16–19.

Bogduk, N. (1997). *Clinical Anatomy of the Lumbar Spine and Sacrum* (3rd ed.). London: Churchill Livingstone

Cholewicki, J. & McGill, S.M. (1996). Mechanical stability of the In vivo lumbar spine: Implications for injury and chronic low back pain. *Clinical Biomechanics, 11*, 1–15.

Cholewicki, J. & Van Vliet, J. IV (2002). Relative contribution of trunk muscles to the stability of the lumbar spine during isometric exertions. *Clinical Biomechanics, 17*, 99–105.

Clark, M. (2001). *Integrated Training for the New Millennium*. Thousand Oaks, Calif.: National Academy of Sports Medicine.

Crisco, J.J. & Panjabi, M.M. (1991). The intersegmental and multisegmental muscles of the lumbar spine. *Spine,* 16, 16, 793–799.

Friedman, P. & Eisen, G. (1980). *The Pilates Method of Physical and Mental Conditioning.* New York, N.Y.: Warner Books, Inc.

Hodges, P.W. & Richardson, C.A. (1996). Insufficient muscular stabilization of the lumbar spine associated with low-back pain: A motor control evaluation of transverses abdominis. *Spine,* 21, 22, 2640–2650.

Jemmett, R. (2001). *Spinal Stabilization: The New Science of Back Pain.* Halifax, Calif.: RMJ Fitness & Rehabilitation Consultants.

Johnston, G. (1994). Living large. *IDEA Today,* 12, 4, 56–59.

Kavcic, N., Grenier, S., & McGill, S.M. (2004). Determining the stabilizing role of individual torso muscles during rehabilitation exercises. *Spine,* 29, 11, 1254–1265.

Krames Communications (1995). *Living in a Healthy Body: A New Look at Health and Weight.* San Bruno, Calif.: Krames Communications.

LaForge, R. (2003). Mindful exercise overview for personal trainers, In: *ACE Personal Trainer Manual,* 3rd ed. San Diego: American Council on Exercise.

LaForge, R. (1997). Mind-body fitness: Encouraging prospects for primary and secondary prevention. *Journal of Cardiovascular Nursing,* 11, 3, 53–65.

Lee, D. (2003). *The Thorax.* White Rock, B.C.: Diane G. Lee Physiotherapist Corporation.

Lee, D. (1999). *The Pelvic Girdle.* London: Churchill Livingstone.

Lutter, J.M. & Jaffee, L. (1996). *The Bodywise Woman* (2nd ed.). Champaign, Ill.: Human Kinetics.

Lyons, P & Burgard, D. (1990). Great Shape: *The First Fitness Guide for Large Women.* Palo Alto, Calif.: Bull Publishing Company.

Melpomene Institute (1996). *Larger Women: Enhancing Body Image, Fitness & Health.* St. Paul, Minn.: Melpomene Institute.

National Osteoporosis Foundation (2004). www.nof.org/osteoporosis/stats.htm

Pilates, J.H. (1934). *Your Health.* Originally published in New York. Republished (1998) Incline Village, Nev.: Presentation Dynamics, Inc.

Pilates, J.H. & Miller, W.J. (1945). *Pilates' Return to Life Through Contrology.* Originally published in New York. Republished (2003) Miami, Fla.: Pilates Method Alliance, Inc.

Richardson, C. et al. (1999). *Therapeutic Exercise for Spinal Segmental Stabilization in Low Back Pain.* London: Churchill Livingstone.

ABOUT THE AUTHOR

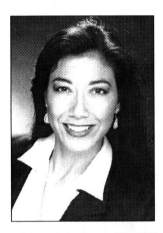

Shirley Archer, J.D., M.A., is a certified Pilates and yoga instructor, group fitness instructor, and personal trainer, and has been a fitness professional for more than 20 years and a wellness professional for 14 years. She is a health educator with the Health Improvement Program at Stanford University School of Medicine. Archer is an international presenter and the author of numerous books, including *Pilates Fusion: Well-Being for Body, Mind and Spirit, The Pilates Deck, YMCA of the USA Mind-Body Exercise Resource Book,* and *The Everything® Weight Training Book.*